Blueprints

Clinical Cases
in Medicine

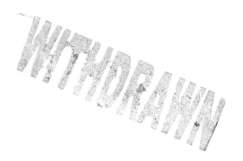
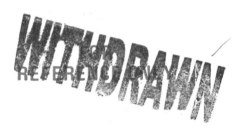
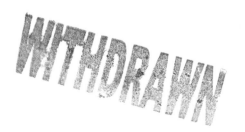
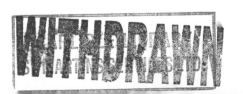

Blueprints Clinical Cases in Medicine

by

Monica Gandhi, MD, MPH
  Fellow, Division of Infectious Diseases
  Department of Medicine
  University of California, San Francisco
  San Francisco, California

Oliver Bacon, MD, MPH
  Fellow, Division of Infectious Diseases
  Department of Medicine
  University of California, San Francisco
  San Francisco, California

Aaron B. Caughey, MD, MPP, MPH (Series Editor)
  Fellow in Maternal-Fetal Medicine
  Department of Obstetrics and Gynecology
  University of California, San Francisco
  San Francisco, California

Blackwell
Publishing

© 2002 by Blackwell Science, Inc.
a Blackwell Publishing Company

Editorial Offices:
Commerce Place, 350 Main Street, Malden, Massachusetts 02148, USA
Osney Mead, Oxford OX2 0EL, England
25 John Street, London WC1N 2BS, England
23 Ainslie Place, Edinburgh EH3 6AJ, Scotland
54 University Street, Carlton, Victoria 3053, Australia

Other Editorial Offices:
Blackwell Wissenschafts-Verlag GmbH, Kurfürstendamm 57, 10707 Berlin, Germany
Blackwell Science KK, MG Kodenmacho Building, 7-10 Kodenmacho
    Nihombashi, Chuo-ku, Tokyo 104, Japan
Iowa State University Press, A Blackwell Science Company, 2121 S. State Avenue,
    Ames, Iowa 50014-8300, USA

Distributors:
The Americas
    Blackwell Publishing
    c/o AIDC
    P.O. Box 20
    50 Winter Sport Lane
    Williston, VT 05495-0020
    (Telephone orders: 800-216-2522;
    fax orders: 802-864-7626)
Australia
    Blackwell Science Pty, Ltd.
    54 University Street
    Carlton, Victoria 3053
    (Telephone orders: 03-9347-0300;
    fax orders: 03-9349-3016)

Outside The Americas and Australia
    Blackwell Science, Ltd.
    c/o Marston Book Services, Ltd.
    P.O. Box 269
    Abingdon
    Oxon OX14 4YN
    England
    (Telephone orders: 44-01235-465500;
    fax orders: 44-01235-465555)

Acquisitions: Beverly Copland
Development: Angela Gagliano
Production: Jennifer Kowalewski
Manufacturing: Lisa Flanagan
Marketing Manager: Kathleen Mulcahy
Cover design: Hannus Design
Interior design: Julie Gallagher
Typeset by International Typesetting and Composition
Printed and bound by Capital City Press

Printed in the United States of America
02 03 04 05 5 4 3 2 1

The Blackwell Science logo is a trade mark of Blackwell Science Ltd.,
registered at the United Kingdom Trade Marks Registry

Library of Congress Cataloging-in-Publication Data
Gandhi, Monica.
    Blueprints clinical cases in medicine / by Monica Gandhi, Oliver
Bacon, Aaron B. Caughey.
        p. ; cm. — (Blueprints clinical cases)
Includes index.
    ISBN 0-632-04603-1 (pbk.)
    1. Internal medicine—Case studies.
    [DNLM: 1. Clinical Medicine—Case Report. 2. Clinical Medicine—Examination
Questions. WB 18.2 G195b 2002] I. Bacon, Oliver. II. Caughey,
Aaron B. III. Title. IV. Series.
    RC66 .G36 2002
    616'.09—dc21
                                                                    2002003530

Notice: The indications and dosages of all drugs in this book have been recommended in the medical literature and conform to the practices of the general community. The medications described and treatment prescriptions suggested do not necessarily have specific approval by the Food and Drug Administration for use in the diseases and dosages for which they are recommended. The package insert for each drug should be consulted for use and dosage as approved by the FDA. Because standards for usage change, it is advisable to keep abreast of revised recommendations, particularly those concerning new drugs.

DEDICATION

To my parents, Om P. and Santosh Gandhi
Monica

To Drs. Redonda Miller, Nancy Codori, and Hunter Young; and to the Osler Medical Service housestaff 1996–1999.
Oliver

We would all like to thank the staff at Blackwell Publishing particularly Bev Copland, Angela Gagliano, and Jen Kowalewski for their untiring work on this project. We would also like to thank our family, friends, and colleagues including the residents and faculty in the Departments of Medicine, Infectious Disease, and Obstetrics and Gynecology at UCSF. I dedicate this book to my grandmother, Elizabeth, who earned her undergraduate degree in her 70s and continues to inspire me with her curiosity and commitment to community service.
Aaron

CONTENTS

Preface   ix
Abbreviations/Acronyms   x

CASES   1

CASES PRESENTING WITH SHORTNESS OF BREATH

CASE **1**   Acute Shortness of Breath in a Young Woman   2
CASE **2**   Very Short of Breath   4
CASE **3**   Shortness of Breath Over One Year   6
CASE **4**   Chronic Shortness of Breath   8
CASE **5**   Hypertensive, Short of Breath, and Dizzy   10
CASE **6**   Fever and Shortness of Breath   12
CASE **7**   Young Woman with Shortness of Breath   14
CASE **8**   White Lungs   16
CASE **9**   Fever, Sweats, and Painful Cough in an Exotic Dancer   18
CASE **10** Fever, Productive Cough, Shortness of Breath   20
CASE **11** Shortness of Breath and Palpitations   22

CASES PRESENTING WITH PAIN IN AND AROUND THE CHEST

CASE **12** Chest Pain, Shortness of Breath   24
CASE **13** Severe Back Pain   26
CASE **14** Syncopal Episode   28
CASE **15** 49-Year-Old Man with Left Shoulder Pain   30
CASE **16** 53-Year-Old Man with Chest Pain   32

CASES PRESENTING WITH PAIN IN AND AROUND THE ABDOMEN

CASE **17** Eating French Fries Hurts!   34
CASE **18** Tarry, Smelly Stools, and Hematemesis   36
CASE **19** Fever, Right Upper Quadrant Pain   38
CASE **20** Diarrhea on the Plane   40
CASE **21** Fever, Diarrhea, and Abdominal Cramping in a Young Man   42
CASE **22** 41-Year-Old Man with Abdominal Pain   44
CASE **23** Hurts to Eat   46
CASE **24** Gnawing Epigastric Pain, Nausea, and Vomiting   48
CASE **25** Too Much Tylenol   50
CASE **26** Fever, Swollen Abdomen, Drowsy, and Yellow   52
CASE **27** Fever, Abdominal Pain, and Foot Drop   54

CONTENTS

CASES PRESENTING WITH A HORMONAL IMBALANCE

CASE 28	Young Woman, Breathing Hard, with Sunken Cheeks	56
CASE 29	Slowing Down	58
CASE 30	Cancerous Calcification	60
CASE 31	Dizzy When I Stand Up	62
CASE 32	Keeping That Sugar Down	64
CASE 33	Jittery	66

CASES PRESENTING WITH PATIENTS WANTING TO KEEP IN GOOD HEALTH

CASE 34	65-Year-Old Woman Who Hasn't Seen a Doctor Recently	68
CASE 35	Calculating Cholesterol	70
CASE 36	Reaction to TB	72

CASES PRESENTING WITH PAIN IN AND AROUND THE HEAD

CASE 37	Headache, Fever	74
CASE 38	Stuffy Nose	76
CASE 39	Fever, Sore Throat	78

CASES PRESENTING WITH TROUBLE IN THE BLOOD

CASE 40	Bleeding Gums	80
CASE 41	50-Year-Old Man with Fatigue and Nosebleed	82
CASE 42	Abnormal Lab Values in a Man with an Abscess	84
CASE 43	Feverish, Bleeding, and Confused	86
CASE 44	New Relationship	88

CASES PRESENTING WITH PATIENTS THAT ARE SWELLING UP

CASE 45	Swollen After a Sore Throat	90
CASE 46	Painful, Swollen Knee	92
CASE 47	Sore Wrist	94
CASE 48	Swollen Legs and Puffy Eyelids in a 35-Year-Old Woman	96
CASE 49	Swollen, Painful Joints	98
CASE 50	Tired of Uremia	100

ANSWERS 103

Case Presentations and Diagnosis	104
Index	139

PREFACE

Blueprints Clinical Cases in Medicine has been designed with several goals in mind. One is to give you yet another opportunity to practice diagnosing and managing 50 of the more common diseases you might encounter as an intern or on step II or III of the national board exam. Another more important goal is to help you to ritualize the process of clinical evaluation itself, so that your findings become thorough, your interpretations thoughtful, and your communication clear, benefiting patients and professional colleagues alike.

Most of the cases in this book describe a patient at the time of presentation to the hospital emergency department. The case descriptions follow the classic order of history (chief complaint, history of the present illness, past medical history, medications/allergies, and social/family/travel history); exam (vital signs, targeted physical exam); and data (serum chemistries, CBC, ECG, and radiologic studies). As such, each case is a brief piece of medical reportage, essentially the on-call intern's admission note up to the moment of interpretation. The reader's task, with some prompting (the Thought and Review questions), is to take that next, interpretive step, otherwise known as the assessment and plan. One very useful approach is to read with a pen and paper at hand, compiling a list of abnormalities or clues that emerge from each section of a case. This list then becomes the basis for the all-important summary ("in short, this is a 65-year-old man with a past medical history of hypertension and a positive family history of early coronary artery disease, who presents with 3 hours of substernal chest pain, diaphoresis, nausea and shortness of breath, bibasilar crackles, and ST depressions in leads V_2–V_4 . . ."), from which the differential diagnosis, assessment, and plan should flow.

The Thought Questions will usually ask the reader to summarize the case and present a differential diagnosis, while the Review Questions that follow the case are designed to explore some of the specific diagnostic and therapeutic issues of the disease in question. For reasons of space, the discussion that follows each review question cannot be comprehensive, but can be supplemented by a thorough reading of any one of the standard textbooks on internal medicine.

Finally, a bit of advice. The most intelligent, well-read house-officer is useless, and perhaps dangerous, if the clinical information that he or she uses to diagnose and manage patients is wrong. While the cases in this book gather and present information for the reader to interpret, there is no substitute for eliciting an accurate history, performing a careful physical exam, and examining primary data (radiographs, smears) with a trained interpreter, when you are caring for a live patient. While very few medical colleagues will lie to each other, most are still learning their craft under challenging conditions, with limited time and increasing caseloads; patients will suffer if their physician too easily relies on impressions and diagnoses given over the phone. As the internist, you, not the emergency physician, radiologist, or consultant, are responsible for your patient's care. Making the diagnosis and starting treatment with information that you have gathered is also a lot more fun than sitting by the phone with an order sheet, acting on the basis of other people's impressions.

Monica Gandhi, MD, MPH
Oliver Bacon, MD, MPH
Aaron B. Caughey, MD, MPP, MPH

ABBREVIATIONS/ACRONYMS

5-ASA	5-aminosalicylic acid	CLL	chronic lymphocytic leukemia
ABG	arterial blood gas	CML	chronic myelogenous leukemia
ABVD	adriamycin/bleomycin/vincristine/ dacarbazine	CMT	cervical motion tenderness
		CMV	cytomegalovirus
ACD	anemia of chronic disease	CN	cranial nerve(s)
ACE	angiotensin-converting enzyme	CNS	central nervous system
ACL	anterior cruciate ligament of the knee	coags	PT and PTT
ACTH	adrenocorticotropic hormone	COPD	chronic obstructive pulmonary disease
ADH	antidiuretic hormone	CPK	creatine phosphokinase
AFB	acid-fast bacilli	Cr	creatinine
AI	aortic insufficiency	CRH	corticotropin-releasing hormone
AIDS	acquired immunodeficiency syndrome	CT	computed tomography
ALL	acute lymphocytic leukemia	CTA	clear to auscultation
All	allergies	CV	cardiovascular
ALT	alanine transaminase	CVA	cerebrovascular accident
AMA	against medical advice	Cx	culture
AML	acute myelogenous leukemia	CXR	chest x-ray
ANA	antinuclear antibody	DIC	disseminated intravascular coagulation
ANC	absolute neutrophil count	DKA	diabetic ketoacidosis
AO×3	alert and oriented to person, place, and time	DM	diabetes mellitus
		DNA	deoxyribonucleic acid
APAP	acetaminophen	DP	dorsalis pedis
ARDS	adult respiratory distress syndrome	DTRs	deep tendon reflexes
AS	aortic stenosis	DVT	deep venous thrombosis
ASA	acetylsalicylic acid (aspirin)	EBT	electron beam tomography
ASCA	(anti-*Saccharomyces cerevisiae* antibody)	EBV	Epstein-Barr virus
ASCUS	abnormal squamous cells of unknown significance	ECASA	Enteric coated aspirin
		ECG	electrocardiography
ASD	arterial septal defect	Echo	echocardiography
ASO	anti-streptolysin O	ED	emergency department
AST	aspartate transaminase	EF	ejection fraction
AV	arteriovenous/atrioventricular	EGD	esophagogastroduodenoscopy
AVR	aortic valve replacement	ELISA	enzyme-linked immunosorbent assay
BE	barium enema	EMG	electromyography
BID	*bis in die* (two times a day)	EMT	emergency medical technician
bili	bilirubin	EOMI	extraocular motion intact
BM	bowel movement	EPO	erythropoietin
BOOP	bronchiolitis obliterans organizing pneumonia	ER	emergency room
		ERCP	endoscopic retrograde cholangiopancreatography
BP	blood pressure		
bpm	beats per minute	ESR	erythrocyte sedimentation rate
BS	bowel sounds	ESRD	end-stage renal disease
BUN	blood urea nitrogen	EtOH	ethanol
CA	cancer	ETT	exercise treadmill testing
CABG	coronary artery bypass grafting	FEV	forced expiratory volume
CAD	coronary artery disease	FNA	fine needle aspiration
CALLA	common acute lymphoblastic leukemia antigen	FOBT	fecal occult blood test
		FSGS	focal segmental glomerulosclerosis
cANCA	cytoplasmic anti-neutrophil cytoplasm antibodies	FSP	fibrogen split product
		FTA-ABS	fluorescent treponemal antibody absorption
CAP	community-acquired pneumonia		
CBC	complete blood count	FVC	forced vital capacity
CD	Crohn's disease	G	gravida (pregnancies)
CFS	cerebrospinal fluid	GEN	general appearance (physical exam)
CHF	congestive heart failure	GERD	gastroesophageal reflux disease
CK	creatine kinase	GFR	glomerular filtration rate
Cl	chloride	GGT	gamma glutamyl transferase

GH	growth hormone
GI	gastrointestinal
GNR	gram-negative rod
GPC	gram-positive cocci
GU	genitourinary
h/o	history of
HAART	highly active antiretroviral therapy
HAV	hepatitis A virus
HBA1C	hemoglobin A1C
HBcAb	hepatitis B core antibody
HBeAg	hepatitis B early antigen
HBsAb	hepatitis b surface antibody
HBsAg	hepatitis B surface antigen
HBV	hepatitis B virus
HCO_3	bicarbonate
Hct	hematocrit
HCTZ	hydrochlorothiazide
HCV	hepatitis C virus
HDL	high density lipoprotein
HEENT	head, eyes, ears, nose, and throat
HIT	heparin-induced thrombocytopenia
HIV	human immunodeficiency virus
HLA	human leukocyte antigen
HPI	history of present illness
HR	heart rate
HRCT	high-resolution CT scan
HRT	hormone replacement therapy
HS	hereditary spherocytosis
HSM	hepatosplenomegaly
HSV	herpes simplex virus
HTN	hypertension
HUS	hemolytic uremic syndrome
IBD	inflammatory bowel disease
ICU	intensive care unit
ID/CC	identification and chief complaint
IDDM	insulin-dependent diabetes mellitus
Ig	immunoglobulin
IM	intramuscular
INH	isoniazid
INR	international normalized ratio
ITP	immune-mediated thrombocytopenia
IV	intravenous
IVDU	intravenous drug use
IVIg	intravenous immunoglobulin
JVD	jugular venous distention
JVP	jugular venous pressure
K	potassium
KOH	potassium hydroxide
KS	Kaposi's sarcoma
KUB	kidneys/ureter/bladder
LAN	lymphadenopathy
LDH	lactate dehydrogenase
LDL	low density lipoprotein
LE	lower extremities
LES	lower esophageal sphincter
LFTs	liver function tests
LLSB	left lower sternal border
LMP	last menstrual period
LP	lumbar puncture
LTBI	latent tuberculosis infection
LV	left ventricular
LVH	left ventricular hypertrophy
Lytes	electrolytes
MAC/MAI	mycobacterium avium complex/ intracellulare
MAHA	microangiopathic hemolytic anemia

MAP	mean arterial pressure
MCD	minimal-change disease
MCHC	mean corpuscular hemoglobin concentration
MCV	mean corpuscular volume
MEDS	medications
MEN	multiple endocrine neoplasia
mgr	murmurs, gallops, or rubs
MGUS	monoclonal gammopathy of undetermined significance
MHC	major histocompatibility complex
MI	myocardial infarction
MOPP	mechlorethamine/vincristine (Oncovorin)/procarbazine/prednisone
MR	mitral regurgitation
MRI	magnetic resonance imaging
MRSA	methicillin-resistant *Staphylococcus aureus*
MSSA	methicillin-sensitive *Staphylococcus aureus*
Na	sodium
NAD	no acute distress
ND	nondistended (abdomen)
NG	nasogastric
NHL	non-Hodgkin's lymphoma
NIDDM	non-insulin-dependent diabetes mellitus
NKDA	no known drug allergies
NPO	*nil per os* (nothing by mouth)
NQWMI	non-Q wave myocardial infarction
NSAID	nonsteroidal anti-inflammatory drug
NSR	normal sinus rhythm
NT	nontender (abdomen)
O+P	ova and parasites
O_2 sat	oxygen saturation
Ob/Gyn	obstetric/gynecologic
OG	orogastric
OP	oropharynx
ORIF	open reduction and internal fixation of fracture
OTC	over-the-counter
P	para (births of viable offspring)
PA	posteroanterior
PAN	polyarteritis nodosa
pANCA	perinuclear anti-neutrophil cytoplasmic antibodies
PBS	peripheral blood smear
PCN	penicillin
pCO_2	partial pressure of carbon dioxide in bloodstream
PCP	*Pneumocystis carinii* pneumonia
PCR	polymerase chain reaction
PE	physical exam
PERRLA	pupils equal, round and reactive to light and accommodation
PFT	pulmonary function test
Plt	platelets
PMHx	past medical history
PMI	point of maximal impulse
PMN	polymorphonuclear leukocyte
PND	paroxysmal nocturnal dyspnea
PO	*per os* (by mouth)
pO_2	partial pressure of oxygen in bloodstream
ppd	packs per day
PPD	purified protein derivative of tuberculin
PRN	*pro re nata* (as needed)
PSA	prostate serum antigen
PSHx	past surgical history

ABBREVIATIONS/ACRONYMS

PSGN	poststreptococcal glomerulonephritis
PT	prothrombin time
PTA	prior to admission
PTCA	percutaneous transluminal coronary angioplasty
PTH	parathyroid hormone
PTT	partial thromboplastin time
PTU	propylthiouracil
PUD	peptic ulcer disease
QD	*quaque die* (every day)
RA	room air OR rheumatoid arthritis
RBC	red blood cell
RLL	right lower lobe
RML	right middle lobe
ROM	range of motion
ROS	review of systems
RPR	rapid plasma reagin
RR	respiratory rate
RRR	regular rate and rhythm
RS	Reed-Sternberg (cell)
RUQ	right upper quadrant
RV	right ventricular
RVH	right ventricular hypertrophy
S_1, S_2, S_3, S_4	1st, 2nd, 3rd, 4th heart sounds
SAAG	serum-ascites albumin gradient
Sab	spontaneous abortion
SBFT	small bowel follow-through
SBP	spontaneous bacterial peritonitis
SHx	social history
SIADH	syndrome of inappropriate secretion of ADH
SK	streptokinase
SLE	systemic lupus erythematosus
SMA	superior mesenteric artery
SMV	superior mesenteric vein
SOB	shortness of breath

STD	sexually transmitted disease
STI	sexually transmitted infection
T_3	triiodothyronine
T_4	thyroxine
Tab	therapeutic abortion
tachy	tachycardic
TB	tuberculosis
TEE	transesophageal echocardiogram
Temp	temperature
TFTs	thyroid function tests
TIA	temporary ischemic attack
TIBC	total iron-binding capacity
TID	*ter in die* (three times a day)
TIPS	transjugular intrahepatic portosystemic shunt
TM	tympanic membrane
TMP/SMX	trimethoprim/sulfamethoxazole
TNF	tumor necrosis factor
tPA	tissue plasminogen activator
TPO	thyroid peroxidase
TR	tricuspid regurgitation
TSH	thyroid-stimulating hormone
TTP	thrombotic thrombocytopenic purpura
UA	urinalysis
UC	ulcerative colitis
UGI	upper GI
URI	upper respiratory tract infection
UTI	urinary tract infection
VDRL	Venereal Disease Research Laboratory
VS	vital signs
VT	ventricular tachycardia
WBC	white blood cell
WDWN	well-developed, well-nourished
WNL	within normal limits
WPW	Wolff-Parkinson-White (syndrome)
XR	x-ray

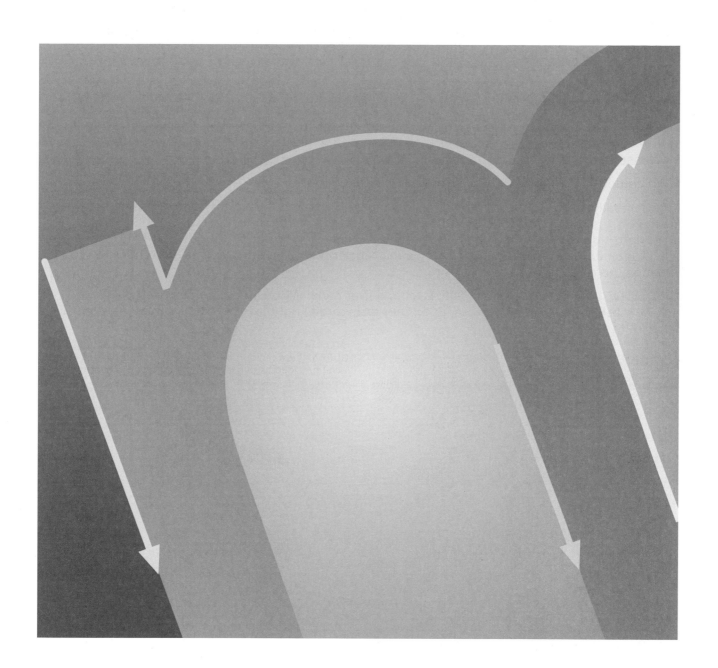

CASES

CASE 1 / ACUTE SHORTNESS OF BREATH IN A YOUNG WOMAN

CC/ID: 39-year-old woman presents with SOB.

HPI: A.G. is a 39-year-old woman generally in good health who presents to urgent care complaining of severe SOB. Also complains of sharp pain in her chest when she takes a deep breath, and anxiety secondary to the SOB with mild lightheadedness. No other complaints—no fevers, chills, cough, trauma, leg pain, or swelling, abdominal pain, nausea or vomiting, diarrhea/constipation, or urinary symptoms.

PMHx: None   **Meds:** Oral contraceptive pills   **All:** NKDA

SHx: Works in a computer technology firm; heterosexual but not currently sexually active; HIV test 3 months ago was negative; smokes one-half to one ppd for 16 years; social EtOH only; no IVDU; occasional marijuana.

VS: Temp 37.5°C, HR 135, BP 102/60, RR 28, O_2 sat 88% RA

PE: Generally anxious, thin, dyspneic young woman in apparent respiratory distress, using accessory muscles of respiration. *HEENT:* OP clear. *Neck:* JVD elevated to ~9 cm; no LAN. *CV:* RRR; S_1, loud S_2; tachy; right-sided S_4; RV lift present. *Lungs:* sporadic wheezing throughout both lung fields, otherwise clear. *Abdomen:* soft; +BS; NT/ND; hepatojugular reflex observed. *Ext:* no edema; no tenderness to palpation; no cords; negative Homan's sign.

Labs: WBC 10.0; Hct 38.0; Plt 210,000; Lytes and liver panel WNL; Urine pregnancy test negative; ABG 7.48/30/68 ($pH/PCO_2/pO_2$) on RA. *ECG:* sinus tachycardia; right axis deviation; otherwise normal. *CXR:* Figure 1.

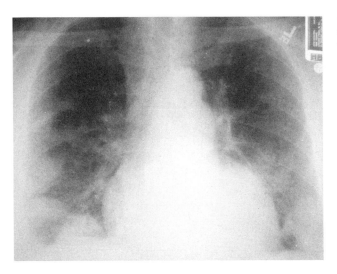

FIGURE 1 Chest radiograph on presentation of patient A.G. (Image provided by Department of Radiology, University of California, San Francisco.)

THOUGHT QUESTIONS
- What is this patient's calculated A-a gradient?
- What is the most likely diagnosis for patient's SOB?
- What are some chest x-ray findings associated with this diagnosis?
- What is Virchow's triad?

The alveolar-arterial O_2 gradient equation is

$$\text{A-a gradient} = 714 \times \text{FIO}_2 - 1.25\,(\text{pCO}_2) - \text{pO}_2$$

At room air, $\text{FIO}_2 = 0.21$

so in this patient

$$\text{A-a gradient} = 150 - 1.25\,(\text{pCO}_2) - \text{pO}_2$$
$$= 150 - 1.25\,(30) - 68 = 44.5$$

This patient most likely has suffered an acute pulmonary embolus, given her sudden onset of SOB without any underlying pulmonary conditions, accompanied by profound tachypnea, dyspnea, and hypoxemia. Physical findings commensurate with this diagnosis include findings of right heart strain on examination, including elevated jugular venous distention, right-sided S_4, right ventricular lift, and hepatojugular reflex. The ABG confirms respiratory alkalosis, hypoxemia, and an elevated A-a gradient. The ECG shows signs of right heart strain with right axis deviation.

The chest x-ray is often clear in the presence of a pulmonary embolus, although findings may include pleural effusion, atelectasis, pulmonary infiltrates, "Hampton's hump" (pleural based density with a convex surface pointing toward the hilum), or "Westermark sign" (decreased vascularity).

Virchow's triad defines the three main risk factors for intravascular thrombosis. The three components of Virchow's triad are 1) abnormalities in the vessel wall, 2) abnormalities within the circulating blood, and 3) stasis of blood flow. Although many prothrombotic states are characterized by more than one defect, profound isolated defects may be sufficient to provoke thrombosis. Patients who present with a pulmonary embolus usually have a defined risk factor for hypercoagulability. The primary hypercoagulable states are caused by quantitative or qualitative abnormalities of specific coagulation proteins that lead to a prothrombotic state. Most of these disorders involve inherited mutations in one of the physiologic antithrombotic factors, and are associated with a lifelong predisposition to thrombosis usually when combined with other prothrombotic mutations or an acquired (secondary) hypercoagulable state (see the answer to Question 3).

CASE CONTINUED

The patient underwent a ventilation-perfusion scan, which revealed a high probability of pulmonary embolus. She was started on heparin and then on warfarin the next day, and was discharged on 6 months of warfarin therapy. Her risk factors for developing a pulmonary embolus were thought to be oral contraceptive pills combined with her smoking and age, but she was referred to a hematologist for further workup for a possible hypercoagulability syndrome.

QUESTIONS

1. Which of the following diagnostic modalities for diagnosing pulmonary embolus can only be interpreted by knowing the pretest probability of the disease?
   A. Spiral CT scan
   B. Pulmonary arteriography
   C. Ventilation-perfusion scan
   D. D-dimer test
   E. MRI

2. Which ECG finding is *not* usually observed with acute pulmonary embolus?
   A. Normal ECG
   B. "$S_1Q_3T_3$" pattern
   C. Right bundle branch block
   D. Peaked T waves
   E. P wave pulmonale

3. Which of the following hypercoagulable states is most often linked to malignancy?
   A. Antiphospholipid antibody syndrome
   B. Trousseau syndrome
   C. Factor V Leiden deficiency
   D. Plasminogen activator deficiency
   E. Westermark syndrome

4. Which of the following therapeutic options for the treatment of deep vein thromboses and pulmonary embolisms does not require lab monitoring of prothrombin time (PT) or partial thromboplastin time (PTT)?
   A. Unfractionated heparin
   B. Warfarin
   C. Coumadin
   D. Hirudin
   E. Low-molecular-weight heparin (enoxaparin)

CC/ID: 36-year-old man with h/o asthma presents to the ER with severe SOB.

HPI: A.D. is a Filipino man with history of asthma since childhood. He has a h/o multiple hospitalizations for asthma exacerbations and has been intubated five times in past. He has had multiple courses of steroids for asthma. He presents to the ER today with a 5-day h/o increasing SOB. He developed a URI approximately 7 days ago, manifested as mild sore throat, coryza, bilateral ear pain, and sneezing. Soon thereafter, he started developing SOB and wheezing, requiring massive doses of his usual inhalers and home nebulizer treatments. He has come in today because he feels like he is getting "very tired" from trying to breathe. A.D. denies any fevers, chills, abdominal pain, nausea, vomiting, diarrhea or constipation, or urinary symptoms. A.D. has had a cough productive of whitish-yellow sputum over the past week. He has sick contacts: two children at home have URIs.

PMHx: Allergic rhinitis; pulmonary TB as child in the Philippines; eczema; cholecystectomy 5 years ago.

Meds: Albuterol and Atrovent inhalers and home nebulizer treatments; flunisolide; Serevent; Singulair, cromolyn sodium; Claritin, Vancenase nasal spray

All: ASA ("makes my asthma worse")

SHx: H/o smoking up to 5 years ago; social drinker; no IVDU or drugs; married with two children; works as medical nurse; has dog at home.

FHx: H/o atopy and DM in family. Mother died of MI age 50; father died of diabetes-related complications age 58.

VS: Temp 36.8°C, BP 110/70, HR 115, RR 40, O_2 sat 89% on RA

PE: *Gen:* unable to complete full sentences secondary to SOB; using accessory of muscles of respiration to breathe; profoundly anxious. *HEENT:* mild pain to palpation over maxillary sinuses; OP clear except for mild erythema posterior pharynx; right TM with erythema, but light reflex intact. *Neck:* retraction present; shotty anterior cervical LAN bilaterally; JVP ~8 cm. *CV:* RRR; S_1S_2 with right-sided S_3; mild TR murmur; no rubs; mild right-sided heave. *Lungs:* very poor air movement throughout; faint end-expiratory wheezing upper lobes. *Abdomen:* soft; +BS; NT/ND; mild hepatomegaly. *Ext:* 1+ edema bilaterally; +clubbing; no cyanosis.

Labs: WBC 7.00 with normal differential; Hct 48.0; Plt 210,000; Na 137; K 3.2; Cl 110; HCO_3 38; BUN 20; Cr 0.9; ABG on RA pH 7.34; pCO_2 59; pO_2 74; *CXR:* clear.

THOUGHT QUESTIONS
- What do the parameters of the ABG indicate about this patient's respiratory status?
- What do his findings on physical examination tell you about this patient's chronic respiratory status?
- What would be the probable next step in his management?

This patient is retaining carbon dioxide (normal CO_2 40) secondary to severe obstruction from his asthma, resulting in a respiratory acidosis. In the setting of acute respiratory acidosis, the pH will fall by 0.008 pH unit for every 0.1 mEq/L rise in $[HCO_3^-]$. However, in the setting of chronic respiratory acidosis, when chronic retention of CO_2 occurs, leading to increased HCO_3^- retention by the kidneys, the pH will fall by 0.0025 pH units for every 0.1 mEq/L rise in $[HCO_3^-]$. This patient's pH profile shows that the retention of CO_2 in this case is in the setting of a chronic respiratory acidosis, as the pH has fallen only 0.06 (~19 × 0.0025) unit points. Despite the elevated respiratory rate, the patient is retaining CO_2 and is unable to keep his O_2 saturation elevated, which means the patient is "tiring"—he is unable to manage ventilation without outside ventilatory support. The physical examination is significant for findings of right heart failure, with elevated JVD, right-sided heave, right-sided S_3, TR, hepatic congestion, and peripheral edema; this patient probably has cor pulmonale secondary to his chronically debilitated respiratory status. The typical obstructive flow volume loop in severe asthma is shown in Figure 2-1, compared to the normal flow-volume loop (Figure 2-2). The next step in this patient's management would most likely be endotracheal intubation and mechanical ventilation.

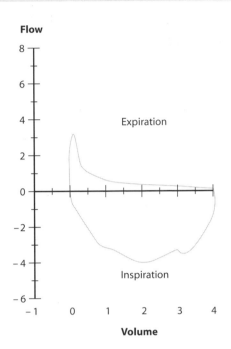

FIGURE 2-1 The concave shape in the upper part of the graph represents the obstruction to exhalation in this severe asthmatic (compare to Figure 2-2). (Illustration by Shawn Girsberger Graphic Design.)

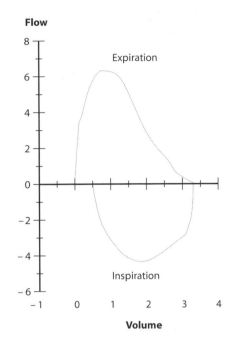

FIGURE 2-2 A flow-volume loop in a patient with normal pulmonary function, showing good expiratory and inspiratory curves. (Illustration by Shawn Girsberger Graphic Design.)

QUESTIONS

5. What is the most likely explanation for this patient's hypokalemia?
   A. Respiratory acidosis
   B. Respiratory alkalosis
   C. Increased work of breathing
   D. β-agonist administration distributing K^+ into cells
   E. Hyperaldosteronism

6. Besides administration of β-agonist and ipratropium nebulizer treatments, which systemic medication should be administered next in the setting of this acute asthma exacerbation?
   A. Cromolyn sodium
   B. Steroids
   C. Theophylline
   D. Leukotriene receptor antagonists
   E. Antibiotics

7. Which of the following is *not* usually a complication of mechanical ventilation?
   A. Pulmonary hypertension
   B. Tracheomalacia
   C. Pneumothorax
   D. Pneumonia
   E. Pneumomediastinum

8. What is this patient's alveolar-arterial O_2 gradient on room air?
   A. >40
   B. Between 30–40
   C. Between 20–29
   D. Between 5–19
   E. <5

CC/ID: 37-year-old woman with progressive SOB for 1 year.

HPI: P.H. had been in her usual state of good health until approximately 1 year ago, when she noted the onset of progressive exertional dyspnea and fatigue. She denies experiencing orthopnea, paroxysmal nocturnal dyspnea, cough, wheezing, and exertional or pleuritic chest pain. She denies using oral contraceptives or cigarettes. She notes a feeling of "fullness" in her neck and thickening in her ankles. After an unsuccessful therapeutic trial of bronchodilators and concern over her worsening condition, her primary care physician sent her to the hospital for further evaluation.

PMHx: G2P2. Appendectomy as a teenager.   **SHx:** Married, two children, travel agent.

Meds: Occasional ibuprofen   **All:** None

VS: Temp 37°C, BP 130/70, HR 80, RR 16, O_2 sat 94% RA

PE: *Gen:* anxious-appearing woman in no respiratory distress at rest. *HEENT:* unremarkable. *Neck:* supple; JVP 16 cm above right atrium. No thyromegaly. Slightly diminished carotid upstrokes bilaterally, without bruits. *Lungs:* clear to auscultation and percussion bilaterally. *CV:* RRR; loud P2; parasternal lift. *Abdomen:* palpable liver edge. *Ext:* mild pitting edema to both ankles.

THOUGHT QUESTIONS

- How would you summarize this patient's presentation so far?
- What broad categories would you include in your differential diagnosis?
- What tests would you like to order?

This 37-year-old woman without history of underlying cardiac or pulmonary disease presents with a 1-year history of progressive dyspnea and fatigue, and signs of right heart failure on physical examination.

Three broad categories of disease that might cause her right-sided heart failure include 1) left-sided heart failure, due to ischemic or nonischemic cardiomyopathy; 2) purely right-sided ischemic heart disease; 3) pulmonary hypertension. Pulmonary hypertension can, in turn, be subdivided into primary idiopathic pulmonary hypertension (less common), and secondary pulmonary hypertension due to underlying pulmonary parenchymal or vascular disease (more common). A partial list of conditions that cause secondary pulmonary hypertension includes: vasoconstriction from chronic hypoxia; loss of pulmonary vessels due to COPD, pulmonary fibrosis, or vasculitis; occlusion of pulmonary vessels by chronic pulmonary emboli or local thrombosis; excessive pulmonary blood flow caused by congenital left-to-right shunting; and cirrhosis, which has been associated with pulmonary hypertension.

Given the patient's age, unremarkable prior medical history, and examination, the likelihood of left-sided heart failure is low, and pulmonary hypertension is of more concern. Nevertheless, at a patient's first presentation, it is prudent to consider the full range of possible diagnoses. Immediate workup should include a chest radiograph and arterial blood gas measurement to look at the pulmonary parenchyma and gas exchange, respectively; an ECG to look for right and left strain patterns and evidence of ischemic damage; CBC, chemistries, hepatic enzymes, and coagulation profile. Subsequent investigation will likely require echocardiography, as well as testing to rule out chronic pulmonary embolism and associated causes of hypercoagulability.

CASE CONTINUED

The chest radiograph shows clear lung fields. There is no hypoxia or hypocapnia on ABG measurement. The ECG reveals sinus rhythm, rightward axis, normal intervals, RVH, and no evidence of ischemic damage. Labs show an elevated hematocrit, normal coags, and mildly elevated transaminases. The patient consents to be admitted to the hospital for further diagnostic workup.

QUESTIONS

9. Pulmonary function testing rules out obstructive airways disease, and both lung perfusion scanning and pulmonary angiography fail to detect thromboembolic disease. An echocardiogram shows an enlarged right ventricle. The most likely diagnosis is:
   A. Pulmonary vasculitis
   B. Ischemic heart disease
   C. Mitral stenosis
   D. Primary pulmonary hypertension

10. Subsequent workup should include:
    A. Right heart catheterization
    B. Chest CT
    C. Coagulation studies
    D. Head CT

11. Appropriate therapy for this patient would include all of the following *except*:
    A. IV prostacyclin via continuous infusion pump
    B. Lasix
    C. PO diltiazem
    D. Warfarin
    E. Beta-blockers

12. Imagine instead that the perfusion scan shows segmental defects and that a subsequent angiogram confirms embolic disease. Further workup could include:
    A. Abdominal CT scan
    B. Bilateral lower extremity venous ultrasound
    C. Mammography
    D. Hypercoagulability workup
    E. (A), (C), and (D)

CC/ID: 62-year-old man with COPD presents with SOB.

HPI: S.B. presents to the ER with a 3-day h/o SOB. S.B. has severe COPD and has been maintained on home nebulizer treatments and home O_2 at night. He has had nasal congestion, mild sore throat, headache, sneezing, and low-grade fevers for the past 5 days and has developed severe SOB for the past 3 days, despite increased use of nebulizers. He has chronic cough, productive of 2 to 3 table-spoons of whitish phlegm each morning, which has not changed. No night sweats, weight loss, or abdominal or urinary symptoms.

PMHx: COPD with last spirometry showing FEV_1 35% of predicted. Peripheral vascular disease.

Meds: Albuterol MDI, 4 puffs QID and PRN, SOB; Atrovent MDI, 4 puffs every 4 hours and PRN, SOB; Azmacort MDI, 4 puffs BID; ASA 325 mg PO QD

All: NKDA

SHx: 90 pack year h/o smoking and currently still smoking 1 PPD; two to three beers on weekend nights; no illicit drugs; former marine biologist; married with 2 grown children.

VS: Temp 37.0°C, BP 125/68, HR 122, RR 24, O_2 sat 90% RA

PE: *Gen:* tired appearing barrel-chested man in moderate respiratory distress, difficulty in speaking full sentences. *HEENT:* OP, no throat erythema; no pain in tapping on sinuses; TMs clear. *Neck:* using accessory muscles of respiration; elevation of JVD to 9 cm; no LAN. *CV:* RRR; S_1, prominent S_2; mild right-sided heave; no murmurs, gallops, or rubs. *Lungs:* hyperresonance to percussion bilaterally and expanded lung fields; poor air movement; no crackles. *Abdomen:* soft; +BS; NT/ND; no HSM. *Ext:* trace pedal edema.

Labs: WBC 8.8; Hct 46.4; Plt 280,000; ABG: pH 7.32/63/68 on RA. *ECG:* sinus tachycardia; right axis deviation; no signs of ischemia.

THOUGHT QUESTIONS

- What are the four stages of severity of COPD?
- Is there any role for systemic corticosteroids in acute exacerbations of COPD?

TABLE 4. Four Stages of the Disease Severity of COPD

STAGE	CHARACTERISTICS
0: At risk	Chronic symptoms (cough, sputum), normal spirometry
I: Mild	Chronic symptoms (cough, sputum) $FEV_1/FVC<70\%$, $FEV_1>80\%$ predicted
II: Moderate	$30\%<FEV_1<80\%$ predicted, $FEV_1/FVC<70\%$ with or without chronic symptoms (cough, sputum, dyspnea)
III: Severe	$FEV_1<30\%$ predicted, $FEV_1/FVC<70\%$, with or without chronic symptoms (cough, sputum, dyspnea), or $FEV_1<50\%$ plus respiratory insufficiency or right heart failure

---

This patient could probably be classified as stage 3 (severe) COPD, given his low FEV in the presence of chronic symptoms (daily cough with sputum).

In terms of the use of systemic glucocorticoids in the treatment of acute COPD exacerbations, this point has been heavily debated, as bronchial inflammation does not seem to play as prominent a role in the pathophysiology of COPD as in asthma. However, the May 2001 guidelines on management of COPD (delineated in the Global Initiative for Chronic Obstructive Pulmonary Disease, or GOLD Workshop Report, http://www.goldcopd.com) summarize the studies on the use of systemic steroids in the COPD exacerbations. These studies overall reveal that oral prednisone, or intravenously administered glucocorticoids, are superior to placebo in terms of more rapid improvement in arterial PO_2, alveolar-arterial oxygen gradient, FEV_1, and peak expiratory flow. Use of steroids in acute exacerbations also led to shorter hospital stays, fewer treatment failures, and a more rapid improvement in dyspnea scale scores.

CASE CONTINUED

S.B. was admitted to a high-level care unit and monitored closely on oxygen and frequent albuterol/ Atrovent treatments. He was started on prednisone (60 mg PO QD), and given a second-generation cephalosporin intravenously for possible bronchitis. ABGs were followed closely, and his respiratory distress resolved quickly over the next several hours. He was discharged after 2 days on a steroid taper, a short outpatient oral course of antibiotics, and follow-up in the Chest Clinic.

QUESTIONS

13. Which genetic defect is known to cause emphysema?
    A. Glutathione S-transferase deficiency
    B. Homocystinemia
    C. α_1-antitrypsin deficiency
    D. Delta F508 mutation
    E. Hypereosinophilia syndrome

14. Atrovent (ipratropium bromide) is in which drug class?
    A. β_2-agonists
    B. β_1-agonists
    C. Aminophyllines
    D. Leukotriene antagonists
    E. Anticholinergics

15. What is the single most effective intervention in treating those with mild and moderate COPD?
    A. Inhaled β_2-agonists
    B. Inhaled anticholinergics
    C. Lung reduction surgery
    D. Smoking cessation
    E. Long-term oxygen therapy

16. COPD is the xth leading cause of death worldwide?
    A. First
    B. Fourth
    C. Tenth
    D. Fifteenth
    E. Fiftieth

CC/ID: 37-year-old man with chest tightness and SOB.

HPI: The patient, a known hypertensive, ran out of his medicines 2 days before admission. On the morning of admission, he woke up SOB, dizzy, and with chest tightness. Too dyspneic to walk, he took a taxi to the ED, where, gasping for breath, he was immediately taken to the acute care area. He is in too much discomfort to give a detailed history, but denies chest pain.

PMHx: Hypertension requiring multiple medications.   **Meds:** Unknown.

All: "Penicillin"   **SHx:** Marginally housed, handyman, unmarried.

VS: Temp 37°C, BP 230/150, HR 95, RR 20, O_2 sat 92% on RA

PE: *Gen:* muscular, agitated man in moderate distress. *HEENT:* blurred disc margins. *Neck:* supple, normal carotid upstroke, no bruits. JVP elevated. *Lungs:* bibasilar crackles. *CV:* RRR, $S_4S_1S_2$, no murmurs. *Abdomen:* soft, NT/ND, no pulsatile masses, +BS. *Neuro:* moves all four limbs; no cranial nerve findings (other than papilledema); agitated, oriented to person only.

THOUGHT QUESTION

- What is your diagnosis, and what further tests would you order?

This patient has a dramatically elevated blood pressure, an examination suggestive of pulmonary edema, and confusion. The most likely diagnosis is hypertensive emergency, which is defined as an elevated blood pressure with evidence of end-organ damage. It requires immediate attention to prevent disability or death. Organs at risk of damage during hypertensive emergency include the brain (intracerebral hemorrhage, encephalopathy, seizure), the cardiovascular system (unstable angina, MI, aortic dissection, CHF with pulmonary edema), and the kidneys (nephropathy with hematuria, proteinuria, and renal insufficiency). Evidence of end-organ damage should be sought with a chest x-ray, ECG, urinalysis, and serial cardiac enzymes. Even without laboratory confirmation, the chest and neurologic exam are enough to make a provisional diagnosis in this case.

CASE CONTINUED

You start supplemental oxygen, place an IV, and take blood for chemistries, CBC, and the first set of cardiac enzymes. You give furosemide intravenously, and nitroglycerin sublingually. There are no ST elevations or significant depressions on the ECG. While the portable x-ray machine is en route, the nurse asks what you would like to do to reduce the patient's blood pressure.

QUESTIONS

17. What blood pressure should you aim for?
    A. <130/80
    B. A decrease in the MAP of 25% in the next few minutes to hour, and then around 160/100 within 2 to 6 hours
    C. A decrease in the diastolic pressure by one-third, but to no lower than 95 mmHg
    D. (B) or (C)

18. MAP (mean arterial pressure) is:
    A. (Systolic BP − Diastolic BP)/2
    B. Diastolic BP + [(Systolic BP − Diastolic BP)/3]
    C. (Systolic BP − Diastolic BP)
    D. (Hydrostatic pressure − Oncotic pressure)

19. Acceptable blood pressure lowering agents in hypertensive emergency include:
    A. Sublingual nifedipine
    B. Sodium nitroprusside IV, with arterial line BP monitoring
    C. Intravenous nitroglycerin
    D. All of the above
    E. (B) or (C)

20. Imagine a different scenario in which the patient was asymptomatic, but came to the ER for a medication refill and was found to have a BP of 220/125 and blurred disc margins on funduscopy. Would you:
    A. Do an ECG and UA, give the patient his BP meds, and monitor him to make sure they worked?
    B. Do an ECG, UA, chest x-ray, and give IV nitroglycerin?
    C. Add a head CT scan to plan (B)?
    D. Chastise the patient for abusing the ER, and refer him to his primary care physician?

CC/ID: 34-year-old man with progressive SOB and fever for 2 weeks.

HPI: S.E., an active IV heroin user, was in his usual state of health until two and a half weeks ago, when the onset of right pleuritic chest pain, fever, chills, exhaustion, and a cough productive of green sputum brought him to the ER. A chest radiograph showing a right lower lobe infiltrate was obtained but never reviewed; the patient was discharged from the ER with the diagnosis of a viral bronchitis, and a supply of acetaminophen. In the 2 weeks since that visit, S.E.'s symptoms have worsened, and he has developed night sweats. He neither takes nor is allergic to any medications.

PMHx: "HIV negative" last year; no surgeries.

SHx: IV heroin; 1 ppd cigarettes for 5 years; social EtOH; sexually active with women.

VS: Temp 40.5°C, BP 110/60, HR 110, RR 20, O$_2$ sat 92% RA

PE: *Gen:* thin diaphoretic man, splinting on the right. *HEENT:* no thrush, normal TMs, PERRLA, no conjunctival petechiae. *Neck:* supple, JVP normal. *Lungs/chest:* tender and dull to percussion at the right base, with egophony. *CV:* RRR, tachy, no murmurs. *Abdomen:* soft, NT/ND, active bowel sounds, no hepatosplenomegaly. *Ext:* track marks on both forearms. No embolic stigmata. Bilat DP pulses.

Labs: WBC 19; Cr 0.6; PT 13 seconds; LDH 90; blood and sputum cultures pending. *CXR:* large, complicated right-sided pleural effusion with RLL and RML infiltrates (Figure 6).

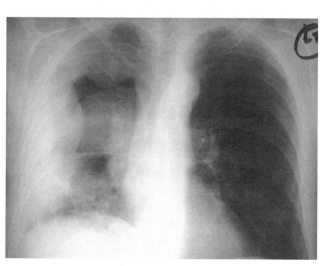

FIGURE 6 CXR: 34-year-old man with fever, sweats, and progressive cough for 2 weeks. (Image provided by Department of Radiology, University of California, San Francisco.)

THOUGHT QUESTIONS

- Summarize this patient's presentation so far.
- What test or procedure will best help you decide how to manage him acutely?

This 34-year-old man, with no known chronic conditions, presents with fever, pleuritic chest pain, SOB, and a right-sided pleural effusion, in the setting of an untreated pneumonia of 2 weeks duration and unknown microbiology. Given the strong likelihood that the pleural effusion seen on chest x-ray represents an empyema (purulent effusion), which would require urgent evacuation, the most helpful diagnostic test would be a diagnostic thoracentesis. The major complications of this procedure include bleeding from a lacerated thoracic artery and pneumothorax from a punctured lung; it is important to rule out a pneumothorax with a chest x-ray afterward.

Analysis of the fluid obtained by thoracentesis allows the categorization of the effusion into one of three broad categories—exudative, transudative, or bloody—that can guide further workup and treatment. A simplified list of conditions that cause exudative pleural effusions includes infections, tumors, rheumatologic diseases (e.g., SLE, rheumatoid arthritis, and sarcoidosis), chylothorax, uremia, and pancreatitis. A partial list of conditions causing transudative pleural effusions includes CHF, cirrhosis, and the nephrotic syndrome. Pulmonary embolism can cause either an exudative or a transudative process.

The most helpful measurements to perform on pleural fluid are of the pH, total and differential WBC count, RBC count, protein, glucose, and LDH. A pleural fluid protein/serum protein ratio of >0.5, pleural fluid LDH/serum LDH >0.6, or a pleural fluid LDH greater than 0.6 × upper limit of normal serum LDH distinguish an exudative from a transudative pleural effusion. Although no absolute number of RBCs defines a bloody effusion, fluid with 100,000 cells/cc appears grossly bloody and suggests cancer, pulmonary infarction, or pulmonary embolism. An exudative effusion with a pH <7.3 suggests an empyema, cancer, lupus/rheumatoid effusion, or esophageal rupture. A low glucose indicates the same set of diagnoses, as well as tuberculosis. In the differential WBC count, a predominance of monocytes suggests malignancy or TB, whereas PMNs suggest empyema, parapneumonic effusion, or pancreatitis. In addition, the presence of amylase is helpful in diagnosing pancreatic disease and esophageal rupture, and cytology is helpful in diagnosing primary or metastatic tumors. Finally, the presence of mesothelial cells is said to rule out tuberculosis.

CASE CONTINUED

Bedside thoracentesis yields tan-colored fluid, with a pH of 7.0, LDH 70, WBC 80,000 with a predominance of PMNs, 1,200 RBCs, and gram-positive cocci in chains. A follow-up chest radiograph shows no pneumothorax.

QUESTIONS

21. Appropriate treatment for this patient's condition includes:
    A. Antibiotics
    B. Serial thoracenteses
    C. Tube thoracostomy (chest tube insertion)
    D. (A) and (B)
    E. (A) and (C)

22. What treatment 2.5 weeks ago could have been prevented this patient's return presentation?
    A. Thoracentesis
    B. Chest tube
    C. Antibiotics
    D. Diuretics
    E. Flu vaccine

23. Imagine a different patient, an afebrile 75-year-old man with known CHF, who lost his medicines 1 week ago and ate an extra-large tub of popcorn at the movies yesterday afternoon. He presents with mild dyspnea, small to moderate bilateral effusions, and pulmonary vascular engorgement on chest x-ray. Appropriate treatment includes:
    A. Diagnostic thoracentesis
    B. Diuretics
    C. Intravenous antibiotics
    D. Sublingual nifedipine
    E. Serial thoracenteses or tube thoracostomy

24. Imagine that you performed a diagnostic thoracentesis on the patient in Question 23 and found a small pneumothorax on follow-up chest x-ray. Would you:
    A. Apply oxygen by face mask and order serial chest radiograms?
    B. Ask a pulmonologist or surgeon to place a chest tube?
    C. Call the hospital's risk-management office?
    D. Give prophylactic antibiotics?

CC/ID: 27-year-old woman complains of SOB.

HPI: A.M. was in her usual state of good health until approximately 2 months before presentation when she noted the onset of progressive exercise intolerance, consisting of fatigue and dyspnea. Three weeks before presentation, she began to experience night sweats, weight gain, and swollen ankles. She came to the hospital today because she was beginning to feel SOB at rest, and had developed a dry cough. She denies fevers, chills, anorexia, adenopathy, headache, chest pain, nausea, vomiting, diarrhea, constipation, or change in bladder habits. She also denies arthropathies, rashes, or change in skin color. She thought she might have had "the flu" approximately 1 month before the onset of her symptoms.

PMHx: Appendectomy at age 12. **Meds:** None **All:** NKDA

SHx: Occasional social EtOH; denies cigarettes or illicit substance use; no transfusions or tattoos; sexually active with men. $G_o P_o$.

FHx: Noncontributory. **VS:** Temp 36.8°C, BP 130/70, HR 100, RR 18

PE: *Gen:* pale, anxious-appearing woman. *HEENT:* PERRLA; OP normal. *Neck:* no thyromegaly; JVP to ears; carotid upstrokes 2+. *Lungs:* bilateral crackles to midthorax. *CV:* diffuse PMI; RRR, $S_1S_2S_3$, no murmurs. *Abdomen:* +hepatojugular reflux; soft liver edge palpable 1–2 finger breadths below costal margin; spleen not palpable NT, normoactive bowel sounds. *Ext:* bilateral pitting edema to knees; peripheral pulses intact.

Labs: CBC, chemistries within normal limits. *CXR:* cardiomegaly, bilateral interstitial infiltrates (Figure 7). *ECG:* sinus rhythm; no evidence of ventricular hypertrophy; nonspecific ST-T changes; no pathologic Q waves. HCG^-.

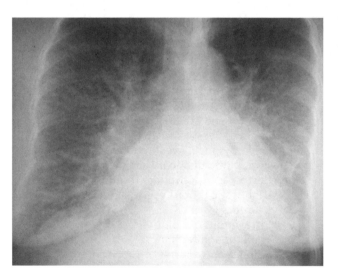

FIGURE 7 CXR: 27-year-old with shortness of breath for 2 months. (Image provided by Department of Radiology, University of California, San Francisco.)

THOUGHT QUESTIONS

- Do you think this patient's heart failure is left sided or right sided?

- What noninvasive test would you request to evaluate her cardiac function?

This 27-year-old woman presents in CHF. She has signs of both left-sided failure (dyspnea, pulmonary edema), and right-sided failure (peripheral edema, hepatic congestion, jugular venous congestion). Right ventricular systolic dysfunction is rarely isolated; rather, it is usually due to left ventricular systolic dysfunction or global cardiomyopathy. CHF is the clinical manifestation of many possible underlying diseases: ischemic heart disease; long-standing hypertension; and any of the causes of dilated, hypertrophic, or restrictive cardiomyopathy. Left ventricular *diastolic* dysfunction can also present with signs of CHF. The presence of an S_3 and a diffuse PMI suggest a dilated left ventricle. After stabilizing the patient, the appropriate noninvasive study would be a transthoracic echocardiogram to assess cardiac structure and function.

CASE CONTINUED

The patient's oxygen saturation on room air is 92%. You give supplemental oxygen by nasal cannula, as well as 20 mg of intravenous furosemide, which produces a brisk diuresis and symptomatic improvement. The echocardiogram shows dilated cardiomyopathy, with global hypokinesis, an ejection fraction of approximately 25% to 30%, and no regional wall-motion or valvular abnormalities. There is no evidence of an effusion. The pattern of myocardial echogenicity does not suggest an infiltrative process.

QUESTIONS

25. The treatment of acute pulmonary edema could include all of the following *except*:
    A. Loop diuretics
    B. Supplemental oxygen
    C. Beta blockers
    D. Nitroglycerin
    E. Morphine

26. Of the possible causes of this patient's CHF, the *least* likely is:
    A. HIV
    B. Enterovirus
    C. Adenovirus
    D. Sarcoidosis

27. The chronic treatment of this patient's cardiomyopathy could include all of the following *except*:
    A. Diuretics
    B. Spironolactone
    C. Beta-blockers
    D. ACE-inhibitors
    E. Calcium channel blockers
    F. Digoxin

28. If the echocardiogram had shown an ejection fraction ≤20%, you would have added which of the following medications to the patient's regimen?
    A. An oral, positive inotropic drug, such as vesnarinone or milrinone
    B. Anticoagulation therapy
    C. Amoxicillin
    D. None of the above

CC/ID: 74-year-old man with h/o coronary heart disease, congestive heart failure, and ventricular arrhythmias presents with increasing dyspnea, nonproductive cough, weight loss, and fatigue.

HPI: P.F. has a long h/o CAD after an MI 3 years ago. At that time, he suffered from ventricular arrhythmias, manifested by runs of ventricular tachycardia, and was placed on an antiarrhythmic with no recurrence since. Also has mild CHF, with a recent echocardiogram showing an ejection fraction of 50%.

Over the past several months, P.F. has noted worsening of dyspnea, manifesting initially with stressful exertion, and now occurring with mild exertion and periodically at rest. He denies any chest pain, paroxysmal nocturnal dyspnea, orthopnea, or peripheral edema. He also complains of a nagging nonproductive cough and chronic fatigue. He denies any fevers or chills, abdominal pain, nausea, vomiting, changes in stool patterns, blood in stool, or urinary symptoms. He has no recent exposure to fumes, gases, cigarette smoke, new drugs, new chemicals, or animals, and has no sick contacts.

PMHx: Hypercholesterolemia. Hypertension. Coronary artery disease after MI 3 years ago. h/o ventricular arrhythmias after MI. Congestive heart failure with recent EF 50%. s/p appendectomy 50 years ago.

Meds: Lisinopril, 20 mg PO QD; Lasix, 20 mg PO QD; KCl, 10 mEq PO QD; Simvastatin, 20 mg PO QD; amiodarone, 400 mg PO QD; ASA 325 mg PO QD

All: NKDA

SHx: History of tobacco 50 pack years, quit 3 years ago after MI; drinks 1 glass of wine every night with dinner; no illicit drugs; lives with wife and has 3 adult children.

FHx: No h/o lung disease in family. Father died of MI at age 66, mother died of "old age" age 80.

VS: Afebrile, BP 150/88, HR 85, RR 30, O_2 sat 90% on RA, 85% with mild exertion

PE: *Gen:* elderly man, fatigued in appearance, no acute distress at rest but clearly using accessory muscles of respiration with mild respiratory distress after moderate exertion. *HEENT:* OP clear; no thrush. *Neck:* no jugular venous distention or hepatojugular reflex; carotids without bruits; thyroid WNL; no LAN. *CV:* RRR, S_1S_2; PMI mildly displaced and diffuse; no murmurs; soft right-sided S_4; no rubs. *Lungs:* diffuse dry rales on inspiration, most prominent in the lower lung fields bilaterally. *Abdomen:* +BS; soft; NT/ND; no hepatosplenomegaly. *Ext:* no peripheral edema or rashes; no clubbing or cyanosis.

Labs: WBC 6.3 with normal differential; Hct 42.0; Plt 320; Na 142; K 4.3; BUN 20; Cr 0.8; Free T_4 7.2 with TSH 1.1; LFTs normal; ABG on RA: pH 7.40; pCO_2 35; pO_2 65. *ECG:* NSR with nonspecific diffuse ST-T changes and Q waves in V_1–V_3, unchanged from previous. *CXR:* Figure 8-1, taken today. (CXR performed 6 months ago was clear.)

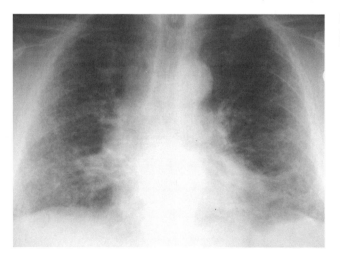

FIGURE 8-1 CXR showing diffuse interstitial reticulonodular pattern. (Image provided by Department of Radiology, University of California, San Francisco.)

The chest x-ray shows a diffuse interstitial process with reticulonodular infiltrates most prominent in the lower lung fields. The differential diagnosis for this process includes alveolar disease from CHF, interstitial pneumonia, or any other interstitial lung disease. Further studies that should be performed to elucidate the diagnosis include an echocardiogram to assess the patient's ejection fraction given his history of CHF, pulmonary function tests to evaluate for the presence of a restrictive lung pattern, and a high resolution CT to evaluate for typical findings of specific etiologies of interstitial lung disease.

CASE CONTINUED

The patient's echocardiogram showed good systolic function with an ejection fraction of 50%, largely unchanged from the previous examination. Pulmonary function tests revealed a restrictive respiratory functional pattern with reductions in total lung capacity, vital capacity, residual volume, and diffusion capacity. A high-resolution CT scan is shown in Figure 8-2.

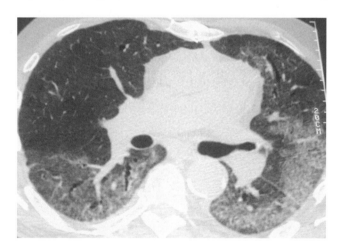

FIGURE 8-2 Asymmetrical, interstitial opacities with a ground-glass pattern. (Image provided by Department of Radiology, University of California, San Francisco.)

QUESTIONS

29. The chest x-ray, echocardiogram, PFT, and high-resolution chest CT findings all point to a diagnosis of:
    A. Congestive heart failure
    B. Chronic obstructive pulmonary disease
    C. Lobar pneumonia
    D. Interstitial lung disease
    E. Cystic fibrosis

30. Which of the following underlying states or risk factors has *not* been associated with this diagnosis?
    A. Collagen vascular diseases
    B. Occupational exposures
    C. Reduction in left ventricular systolic function
    D. Radiation
    E. Drugs

31. Which of the following medications or class of medications that this patient is on is most commonly associated with this disease?
    A. Lasix (loop diuretics)
    B. Lisinopril (ACE inhibitors)
    C. Amiodarone
    D. Statins
    E. Aspirin

32. What is the most common treatment for this particular disease?
    A. Bronchodilators
    B. Diuretics
    C. Antibiotics
    D. Lung transplant
    E. Steroids

CC/ID: 27-year-old woman complains of fever, sweats, and painful cough for 5 days.

HPI: I.E. was in her usual good state of health until 5 days ago, when she noted the onset of fevers, drenching sweats, and shaking chills, accompanied by myalgias and profound fatigue. Since then, she has developed an increasingly painful cough productive of green sputum, and progressive shortness of breath. She also complains of nausea, vomiting, and diarrhea for the last day. She denies headache, visual changes, dysuria, vaginal tenderness or discharge, joint swelling or tenderness, or rashes. Her last menstrual period was 3 weeks ago. For the last 3 days she has felt too sick to support her heroin habit.

PMHx: H/o treated gonorrhea; HIV-neg last year; has no primary care physician.

SHx: Works as an exotic dancer; occasionally trades sex for money or drugs; lives with friend. IV heroin daily for 2 years; one-half ppd cigarettes for 10 years.

Meds: None; denies taking street antibiotics. **All:** NKDA

VS: Temp 40.2°C, BP 125/85, HR 110, RR 18, O_2 sat 94% on RA

PE: *Gen:* bedraggled, uncomfortable-appearing woman, alert and oriented. *HEENT:* OP normal; eye exam without Roth or cotton-wool spots, conjunctival petechiae, or hypopyon; TMs normal. *Neck:* supple; JVP 8 cm from midaxilla; 2+ carotid upstrokes no bruits. *Lungs/chest:* bilateral tenderness to percussion, with peripheral crackles. *CV:* tachycardic, regular; normal S_1S_2; no murmurs. *Abdomen:* soft, NT/ND; +BS; no HSM. *Ext:* scattered track marks on both arms; no peripheral embolic stigmata. *GU/Rectal:* normal cervix, no discharge; no CMT or masses; normal rectal tone. *Neuro:* normal cranial nerves; normal strength, gait.

Labs: Normal lytes, BUN, Cr, UA; WBC 15,000; Hct 38; Plt 300,000. *CXR:* bilateral peripheral wedge-shaped infiltrates (Figure 9).

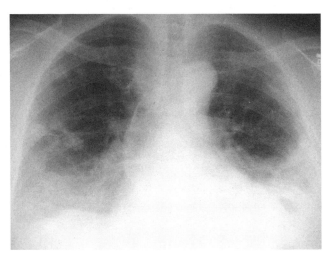

FIGURE 9 CXR: 27-year-old injection drug user with fevers, sweats, and cough. (Image provided by Department of Radiology, University of California, San Francisco.)

THOUGHT QUESTIONS
• Summarize this patient's presentation.
• What additional tests would you order?

This young injection drug user presents with a 5-day history of fever, cough, constitutional symptoms, and multiple wedge-shaped infiltrates on chest x-ray. Her history and examination are highly suggestive of right-sided infective endocarditis with septic pulmonary emboli. Her gastrointestinal symptoms could be a systemic reaction to infection, or could reflect heroin withdrawal.

Serious infections are common in injection drug users. Missing a vein under nonsterile conditions puts the patient at risk for cellulitis, subcutaneous abscesses, and life-threatening necrotizing fasciitis and myositis with staphylococci, streptococci, gram-negative rods, and anaerobes. Successfully entering the vein can lead to an endovascular infection, such as right-sided or left-sided endocarditis, septic thrombophlebitis, or a mycotic aneurysm. Bacteremia, due either to injecting or to embolization from an endovascular source, can lead to metastatic infection involving the eyes, brain, lungs, spleen, kidneys, joints, bones, or skin. *Staphylococcus aureus* commonly causes endovascular infections in injectors, but streptococci, gram-negative rods, and candidal species are also seen. Hepatitis B and C, HIV, and, very rarely, tetanus can be transmitted by needle. Although they are not needle-borne, aspiration pneumonia, tuberculosis, and sexually transmitted infections are associated with injection drug use.

Because of their increased risk of developing a life-threatening endovascular infection, febrile injection drug users should be hospitalized for an infectious workup. This should include three sets of blood cultures 1 hour apart; urinalysis and culture; chest x-ray and sputum gram stain and culture; and a painstaking physical examination to look for occult sites of infection. The importance of performing blood cultures before starting antibiotics cannot be overstated.

CASE CONTINUED

You obtain blood, urine, and sputum cultures, treat the patient's heroin withdrawal, and start empiric antibiotics. An ECG shows no conduction disturbances (AV block can occur if a myocardial abscess erodes into the conduction system).

QUESTIONS

33. While obtaining specimens for culture, which of the following antibiotic regimens would you start?
    A. Vancomycin, 1-gram IV q12h; plus gentamicin, 1 mg/kg IV q8h
    B. Ceftriaxone, 2-gram IV q12h; plus gentamicin, 1 mg/kg IV q8h
    C. Oxacillin, 2-gram IV q4h; plus gentamicin, 1 mg/kg IV q8h
    D. (B) or (C).
    E. (A) or (C).

34. All three blood cultures and the sputum culture are growing methicillin-sensitive *S. aureus.* You decide to:
    A. Treat for presumed tricuspid valve endocarditis with oxacillin and gentamicin for 2 weeks.
    B. Treat for presumed tricuspid valve endocarditis with vancomycin and gentamicin for 2 weeks.
    C. Treat for presumed endocarditis but confirm the diagnosis with a transesophageal echocardiogram (TEE).
    D. (A) or (C).

35. Suppose that a TEE shows no vegetations. Careful examination reveals a tender, warm erythematous area over a femoral vein, which is revealed to be a thrombus by venous ultrasound. Treatment could include:
    A. IV oxacillin for 4 to 6 weeks
    B. Anticoagulation
    C. Thrombectomy if feasible
    D. All of the above

36. While your patient is hospitalized, it would be a good idea to offer all of the following *except*:
    A. Viral hepatitis serologies
    B. HIV antibody counseling and testing
    C. Tetanus booster and PPD (TB test)
    D. Substance abuse counseling
    E. Methadone

CC/ID: 43-year-old woman with fever, cough, and SOB for 3 days.

HPI: C.P. was well until 3 days before admission, when she noted the abrupt onset of extreme fatigue, followed by cough, diaphoresis, shaking chills, and a fever of 101.3°F. Her cough, productive of green sputum, was red-tinged on one occasion and became painful. She took acetaminophen, fluids, and decongestants without relief. When her symptoms worsened and she became short of breath, she came to the ER. Of note, she has been working against a deadline for 2 weeks, and sleeping less than usual.

PMHx: G2P2, LMP 21 days ago. No surgeries. Recurrent UTIs in her 20s, treated with chronic suppressive TMP-SMX; none since.

Meds: Analgesics PRN for menstrual discomfort.   **All:** NKDA

SHx: Epidemiologist with city health department. Married, with two elementary-school-aged sons. No cigarettes or illicit substances. No history of blood transfusions.

VS: Temp 39.8°C, BP 100/70, HR 120, RR 25, O_2 sat 89% on RA

PE: *Gen:* pale, diaphoretic woman in mild respiratory discomfort, A+O×3. *HEENT:* normal conjunctivae; normal OP; TMs clear; no sinus tenderness. *Neck:* supple; JVP 6 cm above midaxilla; no adenopathy or thyromegaly. *Lungs/chest:* dullness and tenderness to percussion at the right base, with increased tactile fremitus and crackles. *CV:* RRR, tachy, normal S_1S_2, no murmurs. *Abdomen:* soft, NT/ND, +BS, no organomegaly. *Rectal:* normal tone; no masses; guaiac negative. *Ext:* no rashes, cyanosis, clubbing, or edema; no arthropathy. *Neuro:* grossly nonfocal.

Labs: WBC 21,000, Hct 37%, Plt 221,000, lytes/BUN/Cr: WNL. ABG: 7.36/40/60/24 on RA. *CXR:* right middle, lower lobe consolidation; no cardiomegaly (Figure 10).

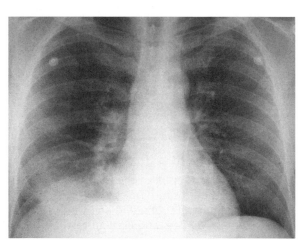

FIGURE 10 CXR: 43-year-old woman with fatigue, fever, and productive cough for 3 days. (Image provided by Department of Radiology, University of California, San Francisco.)

THOUGHT QUESTIONS

• How would you summarize this patient's presentation?

• Does she need to be hospitalized?

This 43-year-old noninstitutionalized woman, without underlying medical disease, presents with an acute illness consisting of fever, chills, productive cough with pleuritic chest pain, ausculatory signs of consolidation, leukocytosis, hypoxia, and bilobar infiltrates on chest x-ray. Although the differential diagnosis of SOB and cough is long, the added presence of fever and lobar consolidation all but clinches the diagnosis of pneumonia, in this case community acquired.

Many patients with community-acquired pneumonia (CAP) can be treated as outpatients, with oral antibiotics. There are several scored algorithms for deciding whether to hospitalize patients with CAP, based on the presence of risk factors at presentation that increase the risk of death. Commonly used indications for hospitalization of patients with CAP include: age >65; comorbid renal, cardiac, or pulmonary disease; diabetes; cancer or immunosuppression; <5000 WBCs; suspected *S. aureus*, gram-negative rod, or anaerobic pneumonia; metastatic infection such as empyema, meningitis, endocarditis, or arthritis; inability to take medication PO; or signs of severely abnormal physiology such as tachypnea, tachycardia, systemic BP <90 mmHg, PaO_2 <60 mmHg; or altered mental status. It is also worth considering whether the patient will receive adequate care at home, and worth remembering that no set of guidelines should replace careful clinical judgment.

CASE CONTINUED

Concerned by your patient's presenting symptoms, you decide to hospitalize her. You give supplemental oxygen by nasal cannula, and intravenous rehydration. Then you stop to consider what cultures to obtain and which antibiotics to start.

QUESTIONS

37. Workup of this patient's CAP should include:
    A. Gram stain of sputum collected before antibiotics
    B. Two sets of blood cultures drawn before antibiotics
    C. Culture and sensitivity of high-quality sputum collected before antibiotics
    D. HIV serology, and testing for *Legionella pneumophila*
    E. All of the above

38. Appropriate empiric antibiotic coverage includes any of the following regimens *except*:
    A. Cefotaxime, ceftriaxone, or a β-lactam/β-lactamase inhibitor, plus a macrolide or doxycycline
    B. Levofloxacin or moxifloxacin
    C. Ciprofloxacin
    D. Vancomycin plus ciprofloxacin

39. The sputum gram stain consists of <10 epithelial cells; >25 PMNs; and 4+ gram-positive, lancet-shaped, quelling-positive diplococci. The culture grows penicillin-susceptible pneumococci. The duration of therapy with penicillin should be:
    A. From the time you switch from proper empiric therapy until 3 to 5 days after the patient becomes afebrile
    B. 14 days total
    C. 21 days total
    D. 7 to 10 days total

40. Which of the following best describes the radiographic appearance of *Pneumocystis carinii* pneumonia (PCP)?
    A. Lobar pneumonia
    B. Bilateral interstitial infiltrates with a "ground glass" appearance
    C. Pleural effusions
    D. Almost any pattern of infiltrate. As many as 30% of patients have unremarkable chest x-rays.

CC/ID: 70-year-old man who presents with SOB for 1 to 2 days.

HPI: A.F. was in his usual state of health until approximately a day and a half ago, when he began to have difficulty catching his breath at rest and with exertion. He denies chest pain, cough, fevers, chills, or leg pain. He complains of mild chest "heaviness," and "palpitations."

PMHx: Type 2 diabetes.   **Meds:** Glyburide, aspirin.

SHx: Drinks 2 to 3 beers at night, more on weekends. No tobacco. Retired long-distance truck driver. Divorced, recently moved in with adult daughter and son-in-law.

VS: Temp 36.7°C, BP 138/80, HR 150 irreg, RR 18

PE: *Gen:* moderately obese man, appearing younger than stated age, in mild respiratory discomfort. *HEENT:* PERRLA; OP no lesions; dentures. *Neck:* JVP 16 cm above right midaxilla; no thyromegaly; carotid upstroke rapid, irregular. *Lungs:* crackles bilaterally 1/3 up. *CV:* irregularly irregular rhythm, normal S_1S_2, no murmurs. *Abdomen:* soft, NT/ND, normal BS, no organomegaly. *Ext:* warm, no track marks, no embolic stigmata; mild pitting edema bilateral lower extremities; palpable DP pulses bilaterally; no calf swelling, cords, or tenderness.

Labs: A PA and lateral chest x-ray confirms mild pulmonary edema. *ECG:* Figure 11.

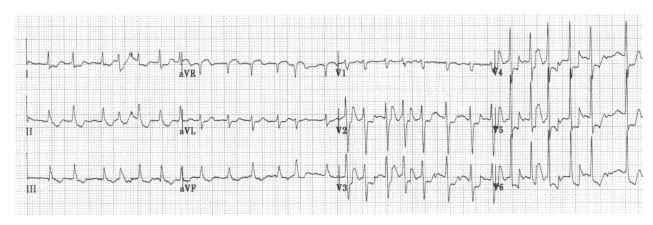

FIGURE 11 A 70-year-old man with shortness of breath and "chest heaviness" for several days. (Used with permission from Taylor GJ. 150 Practice ECGs: Interpretation and Review, 2nd ed. Malden: Blackwell Science, 2002: 184.)

THOUGHT QUESTIONS

• What is your interpretation of the ECG?

• List the possible underlying causes of this abnormal rhythm.

The ECG shows atrial fibrillation with rapid ventricular response and ST depressions that are likely rate-related. The most common cardiac arrhythmia, atrial fibrillation increases in incidence with age, and is often diagnosed in patients without known heart disease. Atrial fibrillation can also arise secondarily due to underlying medical conditions. These include hyperthyroidism, pneumonia, pulmonary embolism, volume overload, hypertension, dilated and hypertrophic cardiomyopathy, ischemia, pericarditis, and alcohol abuse ("holiday heart").

QUESTIONS

41. In the acute treatment of this patient, which of the following therapies would you use?
    A. Synchronized cardioversion
    B. Furosemide
    C. Heparin
    D. Dopamine
    E. Diltiazem
    F. (B), (C), and (E)

42. In establishing a cause for this patient's atrial fibrillation, all of the following tests would be helpful *except*:
    A. Ventilation-perfusion scanning
    B. Thyroid function tests
    C. Head CT
    D. Recent alcohol history
    E. Serial cardiac enzymes
    F. Transthoracic echocardiogram

43. After acute stabilization, further management of this patient could include the following strategies *except*:
    A. Cardioversion within 48 hours of admission and long-term beta blockade
    B. Transesophageal echocardiogram, followed by cardioversion and continued anticoagulation if no thrombus is seen
    C. The same strategy as (B) with the addition of amiodarone
    D. Rate control with diltiazem and anticoagulation with warfarin; no cardioversion

44. After several attempts at cardioversion, the patient remains in atrial fibrillation. He remains symptomatic despite rate control with diltiazem, and he develops pulmonary fibrosis with amiodarone. Which of the following strategies would you pursue?
    A. Increase the diltiazem dose
    B. Switch diltiazem to metoprolol
    C. Radiofrequency ablation of the AV node, and placement of a pacemaker
    D. None of the above

CC/ID: 55-year-old man with worsening chest discomfort for 2 weeks.

HPI: U.A., a 55-year-old contractor, felt "fine" until 2 weeks ago, when he started to experience occasional fatigue, mild "windedness," and left shoulder ache on the job, particularly while carrying equipment to and from his truck. The discomfort would ease at rest. Over the next 2 weeks, however, the episodes became more frequent, and lasted longer before resolving. He ascribed them to occupational muscle strain until this morning, when, while installing a bundle of wires in a ceiling, he experienced an episode of diaphoresis, squeezing left chest pain, and numbness in the fingers of his left hand. The pain resolved after 5 minutes of rest. A concerned co-worker drove him to the ED. The patient can't remember ever having these symptoms before 2 weeks ago. His vital signs are recorded in the triage area. While the ED staff inserts a peripheral IV line, draws blood for laboratory tests, and obtains an ECG and portable chest x-ray, you perform the physical exam.

PMHx: Peptic ulcer disease last year that resolved with a proton pump inhibitor.

Meds: None   **All:** NKDA

FHx: Father died of an MI at age 62, his mother is alive with COPD at age 77. Two younger brothers and one older sister are alive and well.

SHx: Smoked half ppd for 35 years, and drinks 5 to 6 beers/week.

VS: Temp 37.2°C; BP 155/85 (left), 160/80 (right); HR 60, RR 18, O_2 sat 98% RA

PE: *Gen:* thin, anxious-appearing man, AO×3. *HEENT:* PERRLA, OP normal. *Neck:* JVP 8 cm from midaxilla; 2+ carotid upstrokes bilaterally no bruits. *Lungs:* clear, with equal breath sounds bilaterally. *CV:* RRR, $S_4S_1S_2$; no murmurs; pain not reproducible by palpation. *Abdomen:* soft, NT/ND, no hepatosplenomegaly. *Ext:* 2+ pulses in both UE, LE; no cyanosis, clubbing, or edema. *Neuro:* nonfocal.

Labs: *ECG* (at rest, no pain): normal sinus at 60; normal axis and intervals; LVH by voltage; nonspecific ST-T wave abnormalities. No prior tracings available for comparison. *Portable CXR:* clear lung fields, without cardiomegaly or widened mediastinum.

THOUGHT QUESTIONS
- Summarize this patient's presentation.
- What could be causing his chest discomfort?

This 55-year-old man, with three to four major risk factors for CAD, presents with 2 weeks of progressively increasing exertional chest discomfort relieved by rest, and nonspecific changes on an ECG recorded during a pain-free interval. The differential diagnosis of chest pain is very broad, and includes coronary ischemia (angina, unstable angina, infarction); coronary vasospasm; aortic stenosis, aortic dissection, myocarditis, pericarditis; esophageal spasm, reflux, or rupture; peptic ulcer disease or cholecystitis; pneumonia, pneumothorax, or pulmonary embolism; and musculoskeletal ailments. In this patient, the presence of coronary risk factors (e.g., positive family history, cigarette smoking, male sex, possible hypertension), exertional pain relieved by rest, and the progressive worsening of his symptoms are very suggestive for unstable angina. Unstable angina is thought to result from the partial occlusion of a coronary artery by plaque rupture and thrombosis. Such an occlusion can either progress to infarction, or heal, hence the term "unstable." Although he is free of pain at the moment, he should be admitted to the hospital for observation and diagnostic evaluation of his chest pain, focusing on ischemic causes.

CASE CONTINUED

You give the patient an aspirin to chew, and order serial cardiac enzyme levels to evaluate the possibility that the patient has had a non-Q wave MI. As you are starting admission orders, the patient says that his chest feels heavy, and that he is again SOB. You give supplemental oxygen, listen to his lungs (clear), and to his heart (no murmurs), start taking vital signs (BP 155/95, HR 60), and repeat the ECG, which now shows T wave inversions (Figure 12).

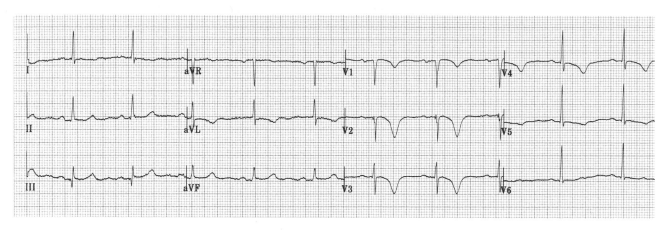

FIGURE 12 A 55-year-old man with worsening exertional chest discomfort over 2 weeks; ECG recorded during episode of discomfort at rest. (Used with permission from Taylor GJ. 150 Practice ECGs: Interpretation and Review. 2nd ed. Malden, MA: Blackwell Science, 2002: 97.)

QUESTIONS

45. This ECG is consistent with:
    A. Unstable angina
    B. Normal variant
    C. Non-Q wave MI
    D. Q wave MI
    E. (A) or (C)

46. Acute, intensive medical management should include all of the following measures *except*:
    A. Aspirin, heparin, and oxygen
    B. Nitrates
    C. Beta-blockers
    D. Thrombolytics
    E. Continuous monitoring of ECG; serial monitoring of blood pressure, heart rate, cardiac enzymes, aPTT, and platelets

47. Proper therapy for patients with unstable angina who fail to respond to initial therapy within 30 minutes could include:
    A. Maximal, tolerated nitrates and beta-blockers
    B. A glycoprotein IIb/IIIa inhibitor such as tirofiban or eptifibatide
    C. Cardiac catheterization
    D. All of the above

48. Which of the following choices best describes the long-term management of patients with unstable angina following stabilization?
    A. All hospitalized patients without contraindication undergo diagnostic cardiac catheterization within 48 hours of presentation.
    B. Hospitalized patients shown to be at high risk for another ischemic event by noninvasive testing, or with a history of MI, receive diagnostic cardiac catheterization unless contraindicated; all others receive catheterization only if medical management fails.
    C. Either (A) or (B).
    D. Neither (A) nor (B).

CC/ID: 65-year-old man with a h/o hypertension presents to ER with severe back pain.

HPI: On the morning of admission, A.D. leaned down to pet his dog and felt a sudden onset of stabbing severe pain in his back. He describes his pain as constant, severe (10/10), and feeling like "my insides are being ripped apart to my back." A.D. called out to his wife, who found him writhing on the floor with pain and called 911. He denies any pain in his anterior chest or SOB, but feels nauseated and diaphoretic with the severity of the pain. He has had no recent fevers, chills, cough, or change in bowel or urinary habits. He denies dizziness, changes in speech or swallowing, but reports pain in both legs as well as the back. No recent trauma.

PMHx: Bicuspid aortic valve diagnosed 20 years ago as incidental finding on echocardiogram; the condition is being followed with regular echocardiograms but no significant stenosis on last study 3 months ago. Hypertension for 25 years, under variable control.

Meds: Amlodipine, 10 mg PO QD; atenolol, 100 mg PO QD; lisinopril, 40 mg PO QD; ASA, 325 mg PO QD

All: NKDA

SHx: Lives with wife; no children; retired policeman; 50 pack/year smoking hx but quit 5 years ago; drinks 6 to 8 beers every weekend; no IVDU or drugs.

VS: Temp 37.0°C, BP 170/110, HR 110, RR 18, O_2 sat 95% RA

PE: *Gen:* diaphoretic, anxious man with pallor and in obvious severe physical pain. *Neuro:* AO×3; CN II–XII intact; strength 5/5 bilaterally in UE; strength 4/5 bilateral LE with reports of numbness and tingling in feet up to midthigh; Babinski's down bilaterally. *HEENT:* OP clear; dry mucus membranes. *Neck:* No JVD; no LAN. *CV:* diminished but equal pulses bilaterally; RRR, $S_1S_2S_4$; tachy; no diastolic murmur appreciated but blowing murmur heard right below the sternum. *Lungs:* dullness to percussion and decreased breath sounds approximately 1/3 of the way up on the left, otherwise clear. *Abdomen:* hypoactive BS; soft; mildly tender to palpation diffusely but no rebound; no HSM. *Ext:* no edema; no rashes; skin clammy; femoral pulses thready bilaterally.

Labs: CBC, lytes, troponin all WNL; BUN 38; Cr 1.4 (baseline 0.8). *ECG:* NSR; LVH; nonspecific T wave flattening and ST changes in the lateral leads. *CXR:* Figure 13.

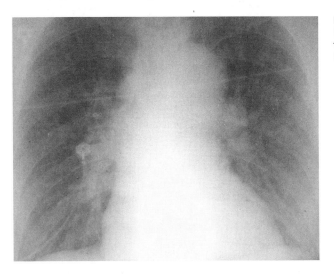

FIGURE 13 CXR shows mediastinal widening. Also (mainly) left-sided pleural effusions in this syndrome can be seen on the chest radiograph. (Image provided by Department of Radiology, University of California, San Francisco.)

THOUGHT QUESTIONS
- What is the differential diagnosis?
- What is the most likely diagnosis?
- How is this syndrome classified?

The differential for A.D.'s symptoms includes myocardial ischemia or infarction, aortic dissection, nondissecting thoracic or abdominal aortic aneurysms, pericarditis, severe musculoskeletal pain, or mediastinal tumors. The most likely diagnosis is acute aortic dissection, given the severity and location of the pain, its sudden onset, the history of hypertension, the presence of reduced pulses, the murmur of aortic regurgitation (the blowing murmur over the aorta on examination), and the widened mediastinal silhouette on the chest x-ray.

Aortic dissection begins with the formation of a tear in the aortic intima that directly exposes the underlying medial layer to the pulse pressure of intraluminal blood, cleaving the media longitudinally and dissecting the aortic wall. The blood-filled space between the dissected layers of the aortic wall becomes the false lumen. The vast majority of aortic dissections occur in one of two locations: 1) the ascending aorta, within several centimeters of the aortic valve; or 2) the descending aorta, just distal to the origin of the left subclavian artery at the ligamentum arteriosum. The classification scheme for aortic dissections defines the location of aortic involvement: one is the Stanford classification scheme, which divides aortic dissections into type A (proximal; ascending aorta) and type B (distal; arch or descending aorta) dissections.

CASE CONTINUED

The patient underwent a contrast-enhanced spiral CT, which revealed two distinct aortic lumen, visibly separated by an intimal flap. This site of the intimal tear is not visible.

QUESTIONS

49. What therapeutic maneuver will offer this patient the best chance of survival?
    A. Cardiac catheterization
    B. Immediate surgical repair
    C. Nitroprusside infusion
    D. Pericardiocentesis
    E. Pain management

50. Which of the following techniques is *not* usually used to diagnose acute aortic dissection?
    A. Aortography
    B. Contrast-enhanced CT
    C. Transesophageal echocardiogram
    D. Transthoracic echocardiogram
    E. MRI scan

51. Which of the following conditions does *not* predispose to aortic dissection?
    A. Marfan syndrome
    B. Hypertension
    C. Ehlers-Danlos syndrome
    D. Trauma
    E. Eaton-Lambert syndrome

52. Which of the following valvular complication is often observed in proximal aortic dissections?
    A. Mitral regurgitation
    B. Mitral stenosis
    C. Aortic regurgitation
    D. Pulmonary regurgitation
    E. Pulmonary stenosis

CC/ID: 79-year-old man with h/o hypercholesterolemia and hypertension presents to the ER after episode of syncope.

HPI: S.V. presents to the ER after an episode of syncope. Over the last few months, he and his wife have been taking walks in the evening in an attempt to exercise more regularly, but S.V. has often felt dizzy and "almost blacked out" during these walks. He denies any chest pain, shortness of breath, nausea, or diaphoresis. On the day of admission, S.V. was walking out the door and suddenly felt "extremely light-headed." After he had sat down, his wife noted that he completely lost consciousness for approximately 10 to 15 seconds, despite her shaking him. He had no preceding head trauma, no changes in speech or swallowing, no changes in gait, and no seizure activity. He denies fevers, chills, cough, SOB, abdominal pain, nausea or vomiting, diarrhea or blood in stool, or urinary symptoms.

PMHx: Hypertension, hyperlipidemia, h/o lower GI bleed 3 years previously with colonoscopy showing arteriovenous malformations in the right colon.

Meds: Lisinopril, 40 mg PO QD; atorvastatin, 20 mg PO QD   **All:** NKDA

SHx: H/o smoking 30 pack years but quit 8 years ago; occasional glass of wine with dinner; no illicit drugs; retired fireman; lives with wife.

FHx: No h/o cardiac or valvular disease in family.

VS: Temp 36.7°C, BP 140/50, HR 80, RR 14, O_2 sat 95% RA

PE: *Gen:* elderly man, thin, in no acute distress. *HEENT:* OP clear. *Neck:* JVP not elevated but prominent *a* waves observed; delayed carotid upstroke with a small, sustained pulse. *CV:* PMI displaced laterally and sustained; RRR; soft S_1S_2. Late-peaking crescendo–decrescendo III/VI systolic murmur heard best at the base of the heart, with radiation to the carotids; S_4 present; no rubs. *Lungs:* CTA bilaterally. *Abdomen:* soft; obese; +BS; NT/ND; no HSM. *Rectal:* brown, heme-neg stool. *Ext:* no edema; cyanosis or clubbing.

Labs: WBC 8.0; Hct 41.0; Plt 200K; lytes, LFTs, troponin-I, all WNL. *ECG:* left atrial enlargement and LVH; no findings of ischemia. *CXR* (PA and lateral): boot-shaped heart; aortic valve calcification on lateral view. *2D-echocardiogram:* concentric LVH; aortic valve area approximately 1.0 cm^2; Doppler reveals mean systolic gradient across the valve of approximately 50 mmHg.

THOUGHT QUESTIONS
- What are the three classic symptoms of aortic stenosis?
- What is the percentage of patients who present with each of those three symptoms?
- What is the implication of each symptom of aortic stenosis for survival?

The classic symptoms of aortic stenosis are angina, syncope, and the symptoms of CHF. These three symptoms form the basis of the natural history of this disease. Prior to the onset of these symptoms, survival in patients with aortic stenosis is similar to that in nondiseased populations. However, once the classic symptoms of aortic stenosis develop, survival without intervention declines precipitously and predictably. The percentage of patients who present with each of the three symptoms of aortic stenosis, along with the time frame in which half of those patients will die without intervention, is presented in Table 14. This study on natural history gives rise to the oft-quoted "5–3–2" rule for aortic stenosis.

TABLE 14. Proportion and Prognosis of the Main Presenting Symptoms of Aortic Stenosis		
SYMPTOM	PERCENTAGE OF PATIENTS PRESENTING WITH SYMPTOM	NUMBER OF YEARS FOR 50% OF PATIENTS TO DIE WITHOUT AVR
Angina	35	5
Syncope	15	3
Congestive heart failure	50	2

CASE CONTINUED

S.V. was deemed to have severe aortic stenosis, based on a valve area of ≤ 1.0 cm^2, presenting symptom of syncope, and the increased transaortic gradient. He underwent cardiac catheterization, which revealed an aortic valve area of 0.8 cm^2 and a transaortic gradient of approximately 60 mmHg. He was referred to cardiac surgery for further evaluation.

QUESTIONS

53. Which of the following is the best initial therapy for a patient with symptomatic aortic stenosis?
    A. Balloon aortic valvuloplasty
    B. ACE inhibitors
    C. Nitrates
    D. Aortic valve replacement
    E. Calcium channel blockers

54. Which of the following medications should be avoided in the setting of severe aortic stenosis?
    A. Digitalis
    B. Beta blockers
    C. Diuretics
    D. Antibiotic therapy for bacterial endocarditis prophylaxis
    E. Aspirin

55. What percentage of the population is born with a bicuspid aortic valve?
    A. 0.05%
    B. 1%
    C. 5%
    D. 10%
    E. 20%

56. What is the name of the pulse characteristic found in aortic stenosis?
    A. Pulsus brevis
    B. Pulsus paradoxus
    C. Pulsus parvus et tardus
    D. Pulsus alternans
    E. Pulsus bisferiens

CASE 15 / 49-YEAR-OLD MAN WITH LEFT SHOULDER PAIN

CC/ID: 49-year-old man presents with increasing left shoulder pain that improves with rest.

HPI: A.M. comes to clinic reporting that he has been feeling well, except for a new pain in his left shoulder and side, which began approximately 2 weeks ago. He thinks it may be related to having been hit in that area during an altercation. The pain comes and goes, and lasts "about two or three minutes." He doesn't think it is related to exertion, although it does get a bit better when he sits quietly. He received a shoulder massage a few days ago, which he thinks helped. Overall, he thinks these pains are "getting better" with time. He denies shortness of breath, numbness in his left arm or jaw, or lightheadedness, and he is pain free at the moment. He is neither diabetic nor hypertensive, and neither parent had early CAD. He does smoke cigars, without inhaling. A fasting lipid profile 2 years ago showed high-normal total cholesterol, with normal LDL and HDL. His physical examination is normal.

Five days later, when you happen to be on call, your patient pages you. When you call back, he sounds anxious, and says that he has been having chest-tightness accompanied by SOB for the last 4 hours. His left arm feels heavy, as do the fourth and fifth fingers of the left hand. You tell him to go as soon as possible to the nearest ED, which happens to be at your hospital. He arrives shortly thereafter; and is brought to the acute room. While the nurses start an IV and obtain an ECG, you perform a quick, targeted exam.

VS: Temp 37°C, BP 130/75 in both arms, HR 90, RR 20, O_2 sat 96% RA

PE: *Gen:* pale, thin, diaphoretic, anxious-appearing man in moderate distress. *Neck:* 2+ carotid upstrokes, no bruits; JVP 12 cm above midaxilla. *Lungs:* clear bilaterally. *CV:* RRR, tachy; no murmur, rub, gallop. *Abdomen:* Soft, NT without pulsatile masses. *Ext:* present and equal pulses in all four extremities; no clubbing or edema.

Labs: *ECG:* sinus rhythm at 90 bpm, normal axis, normal PR interval, ST elevations in leads I, aVL, V_2–V_6; depressions in II, III, aVF (Figure 15).

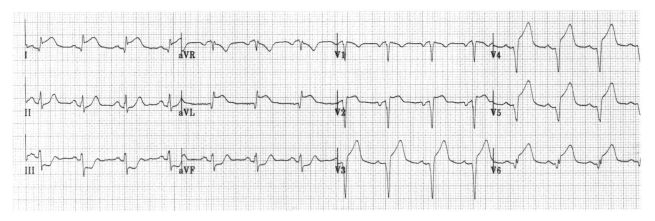

FIGURE 15 A 49-year-old man with chest tightness, shortness of breath, and left arm heaviness. (Used with permission from Taylor GJ. 150 Practice ECGs: Interpretation and Review. 2nd ed. Malden, MA: Blackwell Science, 2002: 109.)

THOUGHT QUESTIONS
- What is the leading diagnosis?
- What were you looking for in your examination?
- What additional information would you like before proceeding with therapy?

This presentation of crushing chest pain radiating down the left arm accompanied by shortness of breath is classic for a Q wave MI. The diagnosis of an anterior infarct is confirmed by the finding of ST elevations in the contiguous leads V_2–V_6. In retrospect, his earlier report of chest pain, although not typically anginal, should have raised the concern of CAD and prompted an exercise treadmill test; it is important to remember that many patients do not describe their symptoms in textbook language.

During the targeted physical examination of a patient with possible MI, it is important to assess the degree of heart failure present; check for mitral valve regurgitation (signaling papillary muscle rupture); and rule out aortic stenosis or dissection. The presence of any of these would alter therapy significantly. Patients with MI and cardiogenic shock do better with revascularization rather than thrombolysis. Aortic stenosis, with its characteristic crescendo–decrescendo murmur at the right upper sternal border, often radiating to the carotids and clavicles, can prove rapidly fatal if misdiagnosed as acute MI and treated with sublingual nitroglycerin. Similarly, finding equal bilateral pulses and blood pressures in the patient's extremities decreases the possibility of missing an aortic dissection, the suspicion of which is an absolute contraindication to thrombolytics.

CASE CONTINUED

The patient denies a history of hypertension, peptic ulcer disease, CVA, bleeding, or significant trauma. You give him aspirin, intravenous nitroglycerin, metoprolol, and heparin, as well as draw blood for chemistries, CBC, coagulation studies, type and crossmatch, and cardiac enzymes. As you work, you decide how to treat his ongoing infarction.

QUESTIONS

57. Which of the following choices describes the appropriate acute treatment?
    A. Continue current medical therapy until the cessation of pain
    B. Cardiac catheterization with percutaneous transluminal coronary angioplasty (PTCA)
    C. Thrombolysis with tPA or streptokinase (SK)
    D. (B) or (C)
    E. (A), (B), or (C)

58. Shortly after starting nitrates, aspirin, heparin, and thrombolytic therapy with tPA, the patient is free of pain and his ST segment elevations have improved markedly. In addition to continuing aspirin and 48 hours of heparin, subsequent therapy and evaluation should include all of the following *except*:
    A. ACE inhibitor and beta-blockade
    B. Echocardiography
    C. Noninvasive testing for ischemia
    D. Electrophysiologic testing to identify inducible arrhythmias
    E. Diagnostic cardiac catheterization

59. The day following thrombolysis, while still hospitalized, he experiences chest heaviness that "is still kind of there" after three sublingual nitroglycerins. Once again, his ECG shows ST segment elevations across the precordium. He is not in cardiogenic shock. Appropriate treatment at this point consists of:
    A. Repeat thrombolysis
    B. Immediate coronary artery bypass grafting (CABG)
    C. Cardiac catheterization, followed by PTCA and intracoronary stenting
    D. Any of the above

60. Which of the following outpatient medications are cardioprotective in patients who have had a MI?
    A. Lipid-lowering agents
    B. ACE inhibitors
    C. Beta-blockers
    D. Aspirin
    E. All of the above

NOTE: Case 15 is intended as a teaching tool, rather than as a comprehensive review of the approach to the patient with myocardial infarction. The reader should study the guidelines for managing acute myocardial infarctions published jointly by the AHA and ACC, from which many of the recommendations in the case are derived.

CC/ID: 53-year-old male presents with acute burning chest pain.

HPI: E.S., a 53-year-old security guard, was in his usual state of health until this evening, when, while napping after dinner, he experienced the onset of "clenching" central chest pain, which lasted approximately 15 minutes and was accompanied by anxiety, diaphoresis, and difficulty catching his breath. It was unlike the "burning" pain of his typical "indigestion," which he experiences intermittently, and which responds to antacids. The pain spontaneously resolved. Concerned that he was possibly having a heart attack, he came to the hospital. Five minutes before arriving, he experienced a recurrence of the pain. On ROS, he denies that the pain was positional, ripping, or radiating to his back. He denies fevers, chills, visual disturbances, exercise intolerance, orthopnea, PND, posterior leg pain when walking, postprandial dyspnea, nausea, cough, hemoptysis, calf swelling or tenderness, or recent prolonged car, bus, or airplane travel.

PMHx: HTN diagnosed 5 years ago, controlled with medication. Sourbrash and epigastric burning for "years." Cholesterol unknown.

Meds: HCTZ, 25 mg PO QD; OTC antacids PRN   **All:** Penicillin ("hives"); denies SOB or wheeze.

FHx: Father died at 58 of an MI; mother alive, age 78; two sisters alive and well.

SHx: Married with two adult children; monogamous. Smoked from age 15 to 25.

VS: Temp 37.4°C; BP 145/95 (right), 150/90 (left); HR 90, RR 16, O_2 sat 98% on RA

PE: *Gen:* WDWN man, anxious-appearing, alert, complaining of 7/10 chest pain. *Neck:* supple; JVP 8 cm above midaxilla; 2+ bilateral carotid upstroke, no bruits. *Lungs:* CTA; no tenderness to percussion. *CV:* RRR, normal S_1S_2; no murmurs, rubs. *Abdomen:* soft, NT/ND, no HSM; no pulsatile masses. *Ext:* 2+ pulses in all extremities; no rashes; no calf swelling or tenderness; no edema. *Neuro:* grossly nonfocal.

THOUGHT QUESTIONS

- What do you think is causing this patient's chest pain?
- If you could order one test, what would it be?

Because this 53-year-old man with new onset 7/10 chest pain, diaphoresis, and SOB has two major risk factors for CAD (male sex and hypertension), an acute coronary syndrome (unstable angina, non-Q wave MI, or Q wave MI) has to be at the top of the list of possible diagnoses. Alternatives include nonatherosclerotic causes of coronary ischemia (hypertrophic cardiomyopathy, aortic stenosis, coronary spasm); aortic dissection; pericarditis; pulmonary disease (embolism or infarction, pneumothorax; pleurisy); gastrointestinal conditions (GERD, esophageal spasm, Mallory-Weiss tear, peptic ulcer disease); or musculoskeletal pain.

Given the high probability that the patient is experiencing an acute coronary syndrome, an ECG is the most appropriate test to order; in fact, it should be performed while you are taking the history and performing the targeted physical examination. Having established that the patient has adequate blood pressure, and having looked for and failed to find evidence of aortic stenosis, it would be safe, and possibly informative, to give a therapeutic trial of sublingual nitroglycerin.

CASE CONTINUED

An ECG, performed while the patient is still experiencing chest pain, shows normal sinus rhythm at 100 bpm, normal axis and intervals, and nonspecific ST-T wave abnormalities (Figure 16). One dose of sublingual nitroglycerin quickly reduces his pain to 2/10; a second dose relieves the pain entirely, and he looks relieved. The ECG, repeated while he is pain-free, is unchanged. He receives an aspirin and an IV line.

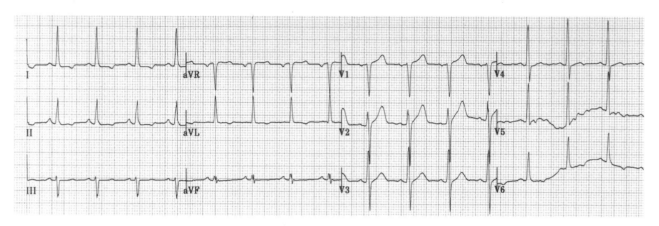

FIGURE 16 A 53-year-old man during an episode of recurrent chest pain; after receiving sublingual nitroglycerin, his pain resolved and his ECG was unchanged. (Used with permission from Taylor GJ. 150 Practice ECGs: Interpretation and Review. 2nd ed. Malden, MA: Blackwell Science, 2002: 162.)

QUESTIONS

61. The most likely cause of the patient's chest pain is:
    A. Aortic dissection
    B. Cardiac ischemia
    C. Pulmonary embolism
    D. Esophageal spasm
    E. (B) or (D)

62. Of the choices listed below, the most appropriate management strategy would be to:
    A. Discharge the patient home on aspirin, omeprazole, and PRN nitroglycerin, with follow-up in GI clinic in 2 days.
    B. Discharge the patient home on aspirin, metoprolol, and PRN nitroglycerin, with follow-up in cardiology clinic in 2 days.
    C. Admit the patient for cardiac catheterization.
    D. Continue to evaluate the patient in the hospital, including a noninvasive test for ischemia.

63. Of the following tests, the *least* helpful for this patient would be:
    A. Serial cardiac enzymes (CK-MB and troponins)
    B. Troponins × 1
    C. Serial ECGs
    D. Fasting lipid profile
    E. Chest radiogram

64. Of the following tests, which would you like to perform first:
    A. V/Q scanning
    B. Barium swallow
    C. Exercise treadmill test with ECG
    D. Upper endoscopy
    E. ELISA for D-dimer, plus venous Doppler studies of both lower extremities

CC/ID: 45-year-old man presents with worsening heartburn.

HPI: H.B. presents to his primary care physician with complaints of daily, severe heartburn, described as severe retrosternal burning pain radiating upward to his neck, occurring 30 to 60 minutes after every meal and continuing for about 4 hours thereafter. Pain is exacerbated by heavy meals, coffee, or spicy foods and is most prominent when lying down at night. H.B. has to prop himself up on three pillows at night to decrease the pain and avoids eating close to bedtime. Also describes an unpleasant sour taste rising in his mouth when he lies supine at night and has awoken occasionally with coughing from regurgitation of food particles. Pain has been worsening over the past 4 months, occurs daily, and interferes with his normal daily functioning ("Doc, I can't eat anything I want to and I'm constantly swigging Maalox"). Mild relief achieved with Maalox or Tums. Only other symptoms are sporadic nonproductive cough and voice hoarseness. He denies any fevers, chills, dysphagia, odynophagia, weight loss, fatigue, SOB, abdominal pain, nausea, changes in bowel habits, blood in stool, or urinary symptoms.

PMHx: Hypertension. H/o subdural hematoma after motor vehicle accident 5 years ago.

Meds: Hydrochlorothiazide, 25 mg PO QD   **All:** ACE inhibitors ("couldn't breathe"); multivitamins

SHx: Smokes approximately half ppd for past 20 years; drinks 6 pack of beer each Friday and Saturday; h/o marijuana use and cocaine use 20 years ago but none currently. Divorced, works in construction.

VS: Afebrile, BP 160/90, HR 85, RR 16, O_2 sat 95% RA

PE: *Gen:* well-appearing, moderately obese man NAD. *HEENT:* moderate erythema in posterior pharynx; mild dental erosions throughout. *Neck:* shotty anterior cervical lymphadenopathy. *CV:* RRR, S_1S_2; no murmurs, gallops, or rubs; *Lungs:* CTA bilaterally. *Abdomen:* soft; obese; +BS; mild epigastric tenderness to palpation without rebound or guarding; nondistended; no HSM. *Rectal:* brown stool, trace guaiac positive; *Ext:* no rashes.

Labs: CBC with differential, lytes, LFTs, UA all WNL. *ECG:* NSR; no ST-T abnormalities. *CXR:* normal.

THOUGHT QUESTIONS
- What is the medical term for the common medical complaint of heartburn?
- What is the pathophysiologic basis of this condition?
- What are some of the methods used to diagnose this condition?

H.B. describes the symptoms of gastroesophageal reflux disease (GERD), a condition affecting an estimated 25% to 35% of the U.S. population, with as many as 10% of Americans experiencing episodes of heartburn on a daily basis. GERD is a multifactorial problem usually involving disruptions in the physiology of the lower esophageal sphincter (LES). The LES maintains a pressure barrier between the stomach and the esophagus and its tone is modulated by hormonal, neural, and dietary factors. Irritant action of acid and digestive enzymes, decreased secondary peristalsis, defective mucosal resistance to caustic liquids, impaired esophageal clearance of acid, and delayed gastric emptying have all been implicated in altering LES tone. In many patients, reflux occurs as a result of transient episodes of inappropriate sphincter relaxation rather than low basal tone. Although the diagnosis is usually made clinically, ambulatory pH monitoring is generally considered the diagnostic gold standard for patients with GERD. A pH monitor is placed in the esophagus above the lower esophageal sphincter, and the pH is recorded periodically. Over the 24-hour test period, the patient writes down the time in which symptoms occur, to ascertain if symptomology can be correlated with the lowering of esophageal pH that occurs with reflux. Endoscopy is useful for diagnosing some of the complications of GERD and can detect an anatomic explanation for the disease (e.g., hiatal hernia) but is not sensitive for the diagnosis of GERD itself. Only 50% of patients with GERD manifest macroscopic evidence of this condition on endoscopy.

CASE CONTINUED

Given the severity of the patient's symptoms, H.B. underwent ambulatory pH monitoring, which confirmed lowering of esophageal pH with reflux symptoms. He also underwent an upper endoscopy (Figure 17) to rule out complications of GERD.

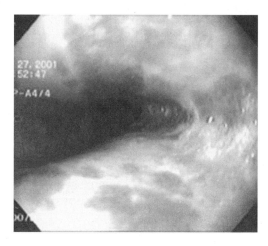

FIGURE 17 Patchy erythema and inflammation consistent with severe reflux disease. (Copyrighted material is used with permission of the author, the University of Iowa and Virtual Hospital, www.vh.org.)

QUESTIONS

65. Of the following factors, which have *not* been implicated in exacerbating the symptoms of GERD?
    A. Exercise
    B. Tobacco
    C. Peppermint
    D. Pregnancy
    E. Foods high in protein

66. GERD increases the risk for the following malignancy of the esophagus:
    A. Squamous cell carcinoma
    B. Lymphoma
    C. Adenocarcinoma
    D. Carcinoid syndrome
    E. GERD is not associated with malignancy

67. The first modality of treatment for GERD is:
    A. H_2-receptor blockers
    B. Antacids
    C. Proton pump inhibitors
    D. Surgical management
    E. Lifestyle modification

68. Which of the following agents has been shown to provide better symptom control, esophageal healing, and maintenance of remission in GERD than the others?
    A. H_2-receptor blockers
    B. Sodium-bicarbonate
    C. Prokinetic agents
    D. Proton pump inhibitors
    E. Magnesium–aluminum combinations

CC/ID: 55-year-old woman who vomited bright red blood presents to the ED.

HPI: Two days before admission, G.B. noted the onset of dull, gnawing epigastric pain that was somewhat improved by PO intake. One day before admission, she had two "black" sticky stools that smelled unusual. The morning of admission, she vomited a "cupful" of bright red blood, felt light-headed, and called an ambulance. She denies fevers, chills, sweats, retching prior to her episode of hematemesis, cramping, diarrhea, abdominal swelling, or recent nosebleeds. She denies unintentional weight loss, dysphagia, odynophagia, chest pain, or a history of jaundice.

PMHx: No known history of chronic liver disease, cancer, or colitis; "threw her back out" 2 weeks ago, and was taking NSAIDs; hypertension; hypercholesterolemia; postmenopausal; mitral prolapse.

Meds: HCTZ, 25 mg PO QD; simvastatin, 40 mg PO QD; ibuprofen, 600 mg PO TID; HRT; amoxicillin PRN for dental procedures.

All: NKDA

SHx: No history of tobacco use, occasional social EtOH; astronomer, married, no children.

VS: Temp 37.5°C; BP 110/80 (seated), 105/80 (standing); HR 100 (seated), 109 (standing); RR 16, O_2 sat 99% RA

PE: *Gen:* concerned, calm, diaphoretic woman in NAD; does not appear chronically ill. *HEENT:* nasal turbinates, oropharynx clear. *Neck:* supple, no thyromegaly. Normal carotid upstroke without bruits. JVP flat. *Lungs:* clear. *CV:* RRR tachy, normal S_1S_2 with midsystolic click. *Abdomen:* soft, ND, +BS. Mid-epigastric tenderness to deep palpation. No HSM or bulging flanks. *Ext:* warm, well perfused, 2+ DP pulses bilaterally. 16-gauge IV line in right antecubital fossa. *Neuro:* AO×3; strength, sensation, and cranial nerves normal. *Skin:* no rashes or spider hemangiomas.

THOUGHT QUESTIONS
- How would you summarize this patient's presentation?
- Where do you think the blood is coming from?

This 55-year-old woman presents 2 days after the onset of gnawing epigastric pain, with two episodes of melena, followed by one episode of hematemesis, in the setting of NSAID use and evidence of mild orthostasis. Defining the names given to the different ways in which a GI bleed can present helps locate the source of the blood. *Hematemesis*, the vomiting of blood, whether bright red, maroon, brown, or coffee-ground appearance, signals a source above the ligament of Treitz (i.e., an upper GI bleed). *Melena*, the passage of tarry, black, sticky stools, usually signifies a source above the jejunum (again, an upper GI bleed). If transit time through the bowel is slow, melena can be associated with a source in the distal small bowel or ascending colon. *Hematochezia*, the passage of bright red blood from the rectum, usually signifies a source distal to the ligament of Treitz, but can be seen in a brisk upper GI bleed. The presence of melena and hematemesis in this patient point to a source in the upper GI tract.

CASE CONTINUED

Someone puts a central line kit in your hand, and asks if you want the patient to have KUB films or a CT scan.

QUESTIONS

69. You reply:
    A. "No thanks. Call the surgeons."
    B. "No thanks. Let's get another 16-gauge peripheral in, send off some blood for CBC, coags, lytes, and type and cross, and get set up for nasogastric (NG) lavage."
    C. "Great. As soon as we have a clean triple lumen in her neck, let's get a CBC, coags, lytes, and type and cross, pull that peripheral line out of her arm, and get a chest x-ray along with the KUB to confirm proper line placement. Then we'll do an NG lavage."
    D. "Who's on call for GI tonight?"

70. NG lavage is useful for:
    A. Preparing the stomach for esophagogastro-duodenoscopy (EGD)
    B. Determining the activity of the bleed
    C. Stopping the bleed
    D. (A) and (B)
    E. None of the above. It is archaic medical lore and should not delay the EGD, which is diagnostic and therapeutic.

71. The initial hematocrit comes back as 37. You should order the next one:
    A. Immediately—the first one is a lab error.
    B. In 3 hours, and every 3 to 6 hours after that.
    C. With tomorrow's morning lab draw.
    D. No further blood draws are necessary.

72. If the patient had presented with 24 hours of melena only, followed by one episode of hematochezia rather than hematemesis, your first move would be to insert two large-bore IV lines, check serial hematocrits, and:
    A. Prepare for colonoscopy.
    B. Perform NG lavage and prep for colonoscopy.
    C. Order a tagged red blood cell bleeding scan.
    D. Perform NG lavage and order mesenteric angiography.

CC/ID: 37-year-old woman with acute onset of fever and RUQ pain.

HPI: A.C. was in her usual good state of health until shortly after lunch today, when she experienced the acute onset of severe RUQ pain, nausea, and subjective fever. She vomited several times, with partial, temporary relief. The pain is unrelated to body position and radiates to the right scapula. Her husband brought her to the ED because she could not stand the pain, which was "worse than childbirth" and wasn't responding to Pepto-Bismol and acetaminophen. She denies any significant prior medical history, or symptoms preceding her current illness. She denies headache, visual changes, chest pain, shortness of breath, cough, diarrhea, rashes, or joint pain.

Meds: Analgesics PRN   **All:** NKDA   **POb/GynHx:** G2P2

SHx: Married, with two adolescent children. Occasional wine with dinner; no cigarettes; no illicit substances.

FHx: Noncontributory.   **VS:** Temp 100.7°F, BP 140/90, HR 100, RR 18

PE: *Gen:* mildly overweight woman in pain, alert and conversant. *HEENT:* anicteric sclerae. *Lungs:* CTA bilateral. *CV:* RRR, normal S$_1$S$_2$, midsystolic click; no murmurs. *Abdomen:* tender RUQ with rebound and muscle guarding. Tenderness increased with inspiration during deep palpation of the RUQ (+Murphy sign). Hypoactive bowel sounds. *Rectal:* normal tone, guaiac negative. *Ext:* no rashes, livedo reticularis, or arthropathy. Warm and well-perfused. Skin tenting. Absence of axillary sweat.

THOUGHT QUESTIONS

- How would you summarize this patient's presentation?
- What would you include in the differential diagnosis?
- What tests would you perform to guide further treatment?

This 37-year-old woman without significant past medical history presents with fever and acute RUQ pain radiating to the ipsilateral scapula, rebound tenderness, a positive Murphy sign, and signs of dehydration. The differential diagnosis includes acute events in the abdomen or right chest: gall bladder disease; liver abscess or hepatitis; pancreatitis; perforated peptic ulcer; appendicitis; aortic dissection; or right-sided pneumonia. The most likely diagnosis is acute cholecystitis, or inflammation of the gallbladder. This is usually due to obstruction of the cystic duct by a stone, although it can be acalculous (i.e., without a stone), or can result from anatomic or functional abnormalities of the cystic duct. The constellation of acute RUQ pain, fever, and leukocytosis suggests the diagnosis. Nausea, vomiting, jaundice, mild hyperbilirubinemia, elevated alkaline phosphatase, elevated amylase, and mild transaminitis may also be present. An ultrasound showing cystic duct stones, pericholecystic fluid, and gallbladder wall thickening helps to confirm the diagnosis. If this is equivocal, a hepatobiliary nuclear medicine scan (or ^{99m}Tc-HIDA) showing cystic duct obstruction (radionuclide visualization of the biliary ducts without the gallbladder) is also confirmatory.

The initial workup of this patient should include CBC with differential, serum chemistries, liver panel, amylase, coags, and RUQ ultrasound with or without a ^{99m}Tc-HIDA scan. Blood cultures would not be unreasonable, given the possibility of cholangitis and bacteremia. If initial imaging studies are unrevealing, endoscopic retrograde cholangiopancreatography (ERCP) and abdominal CT scanning should be considered.

CASE CONTINUED

Labs show a WBC count of 14,000, mildly elevated transaminases and alkaline phosphatase, a total bilirubin of 4.0, and normal coagulation studies, amylase and albumin. RUQ ultrasonography shows numerous stones in the gallbladder and one in the cystic duct, with gallbladder wall thickening and pericholecystic fluid. Two sets of blood cultures are incubating.

QUESTIONS

73. In this patient, proper initial therapy consists of:
    A. Open cholecystectomy
    B. Laparoscopic cholecystectomy
    C. NPO, peripheral nutrition, analgesia, and antibiotics
    D. Cholecystostomy (percutaneous drainage)

74. In this patient, definitive therapy consists of:
    A. ERCP
    B. Laparoscopic cholecystectomy
    C. NPO, peripheral nutrition, analgesia, and antibiotics
    D. Cholecystostomy (percutaneous drainage)

75. Several days after being stabilized, the patient suddenly becomes severely ill, with jaundice, high fever, rigors, and confusion. Her RUQ pain worsens, and her bilirubin, transaminases, alkaline phosphatase, and WBC rise precipitously. This syndrome is called:
    A. Austrian's triad
    B. Osler's triad
    C. Charcot's triad
    D. Jones criteria

76. The approach to this condition includes:
    A. Blood cultures, antibiotics, and ERCP with sphincterotomy and stone removal, followed by cholecystectomy
    B. Cholecystectomy
    C. Antibiotics and analgesia
    D. Exploratory laparotomy

CC/ID: 30-year-old woman traveler presents with bloody diarrhea.

HPI: B.D. was generally in good health until she presented to the ER with a 4-day complaint of bloody diarrhea, abdominal cramping, fever, and profound weakness. She had been traveling through Spain the week prior to admission and started developing symptoms approximately 4 days into her trip. First symptoms were fevers and chills, followed by lower abdominal cramping, fatigue, and diarrhea. The diarrhea is described as moderate volume but explosive, occurring approximately 8 to 10 times per day, with streaks of blood and moderate amounts of yellow-green mucus. She also reports severe nausea with vomiting, usually dry heaves. B.D. has had a poor appetite and has tried to force liquid intake, with very little solid food intake for the past 4 days. On the airplane flight home, B.D. made about 15 trips to the bathroom in 6 hours, having small volume, bloody diarrhea, or episodes of vomiting. She has tenesmus and abdominal pain, which is somewhat relieved with defecation, as well as dizziness with standing, mild SOB, and profound weakness. Patient continues to have fevers/chills, but no night sweats, and came straight to the ER from the airport for evaluation. She has no cough, dysuria, or vaginal discharge, her LMP was 3 weeks ago, and her traveling companion is not ill.

PMHx: Depression   **Meds:** Celexa, 20 mg PO QD   **All:** NKDA

SHx: No smoking, minimal EtOH, no drugs. Heterosexual with one male partner, with whom patient uses condoms. Works as a physician.

VS: 38.4°C; BP 95/60 (sitting), 85/40 (standing); HR 105 (sitting), 120 (standing); RR 16

PE: *Gen:* ill appearing, pale, fatigued young woman. *HEENT:* sunken eyes; dry mucus membranes. *Neck:* no LAN. *CV:* RRR, S$_1$S$_2$; tachy; no murmurs, gallops, or rubs. *Lungs:* CTA bilaterally. *Abdomen:* soft; BS hyperactive; diffusely tender to palpation most pronounced in bilateral lower quadrants without rebound; +voluntary guarding; mildly distended. *Rectal:* bloody green mucus (guaiac positive). *Ext:* skin tenting; no edema, joint effusions or rashes.

Labs: WBC 12.00; Hct 44.0; Plt 317; Na 149; K 3.0; HCO3 27; Cl 98; BUN 30; Cr 0.8

THOUGHT QUESTIONS

- What is this patient's differential diagnosis?
- What clues in the history/physical are more suggestive of a specific infection?
- What is the best way to make the diagnosis?
- How should this patient be managed initially?
- How may the specific travel history change your initial management?

This patient's differential diagnosis for traveler's diarrhea includes bacterial causes, either from enterotoxigenic, enteroinvasive or enterohemorrhagic *E. coli, Shigella, Campylobacter jejuni, Salmonella, Yersinia enterocolitica, Aeromonas hydrophilia,* or *Plesiomonas shigelloides.* Diarrheal illnesses with short incubation periods are usually toxin-mediated and include toxins from *Staphylococcus aureus,* toxigenic *E. coli, Clostridium perfringens, Bacillus cereus,* and *Vibrio parahaemolyticus,* although these illnesses are usually self-limited. Parasitic causes include *Giardia lamblia, Entamoeba histolytica,* and *Cryptosporidium.* Viral causes include Norwalk virus and rotavirus. The history of the relatively short duration of symptoms, fever, bloody stools with mucus, small to moderate volume but frequent stools, and abdominal cramping all point to a bacterial cause, most likely resulting from mucosal invasion. The best way to make the diagnosis in this case is stool culture, with specification to the microbiology lab to look for the suspected bacterial pathogens. Methylene blue staining to look for fecal leukocytes is rarely useful, as the blood and mucus reported in the stool already suggests an inflammatory diarrheal process. This patient has signs and symptoms of dehydration and should be aggressively rehydrated with IV fluids given her inability to keep orally hydrated. After collecting stool for culture, this patient can be started on an antibacterial known to cover the suspected organisms. Ampicillin and Bactrim were former mainstays of therapy for bacterial diarrhea, although increasing resistance among all the agents has been reported; ciprofloxacin is now more commonly used as initial therapy for traveler's diarrhea, but specific regions have reported increasing resistance of bacterial pathogens even to fluoroquinolones.

CASE CONTINUED

In the ED, B.D. was rehydrated with 2 liters of normal saline, her stool was sent for culture, and she was started on ciprofloxacin (500 mg PO BID × 5 days). In 2 days, the stool culture grew out comma-shaped, gram negative bacilli.

QUESTIONS

77. The cause of this patient's diarrhea is most likely:
    A. *Escherichia coli*
    B. *Salmonella*
    C. *Shigella*
    D. *Entamoeba histolytica*
    E. *Campylobacter jejuni*

78. Which of the following measures is *not* recommended to reduce the incidence of traveler's diarrhea?
    A. Drinking only boiled or treated water
    B. Avoiding ice
    C. Prophylactic antibiotics
    D. Peeling fruits
    E. Eating hot foods

79. Which of the following causes of traveler's diarrhea is most commonly associated with drinking from freshwater streams?
    A. Norwalk virus
    B. *Giardia lamblia*
    C. *Shigella*
    D. Enterohemorrhagic *E. coli*
    E. *Yersinia enterocolitica*

80. What is the treatment of choice for the fluoroquinolone-resistant agents of bacterial diarrhea?
    A. Trimethoprim-sulfamethoxazole
    B. Amoxicillin
    C. Ciprofloxacin
    D. Metronidazole
    E. Azithromycin

CC/ID: 21-year-old male has had fever, diarrhea, and abdominal cramping for 2 weeks.

HPI: I.B. is a college student in previously good health, who comes to clinic because of 2 weeks of crampy abdominal pain, tenesmus, and occasionally bloody diarrhea three to four times per day. Defecating relieves his tenesmus and pain temporarily. He has been intermittently febrile to 38.4°C. Since the syndrome began, he has felt more fatigued, and has been taking daytime naps, which is not customary for him. He denies headache, eye pain, visual changes, SOB, cough, chest pain, or back or joint pain. He came to clinic today because his symptoms have not abated on their own.

He has never traveled outside of the U.S., has not eaten any suspicious food, does not spend time in the wilderness, and is not currently sexually active. He has no history of chronic diarrhea or constipation. His past medical history is significant for an appendectomy at age 12.

Meds: Pepto-Bismol, Maalox, acetaminophen.   **All:** Penicillin leads to a truncal rash.

SHx: Occasional cigarette; social EtOH; 0/4 on CAGE questionnaire.

FHx: Father with chronic abdominal pain.

VS: Temp 38.1°C, BP 140/85, HR 77, RR 14, O_2 sat 99% on RA

PE: *Gen:* normally developed young man in NAD, but uneasy. *HEENT:* Oropharynx no aphthous ulcers; normal conjunctivae and sclerae. PERRLA; no sinus tenderness; TMs normal. *Neck:* supple, JVP 8 cm above midaxillary line; no thyromegaly or adenopathy. *Lungs:* clear bilaterally. *CV:* RRR; normal S_1S_2; no murmurs. *Abdomen:* soft; +BS; moderate tenderness to deep palpation in bilateral lower quadrants no rebound; no HSM. *Rectal:* normal tone; no masses; smooth, NT prostate; guaiac-positive brown stool. *Ext:* no rashes, ulcers, cyanosis, discoloration, clubbing, arthropathy, or edema. *Neuro:* nonfocal.

Labs: WBC 8000; Hct 37%; Plt 270,000. Bilis, transaminases, alk phos, PT/PTT normal.

THOUGHT QUESTIONS
- Summarize this patient's presentation.
- What is the differential diagnosis of his abdominal syndrome?
- What is the most likely diagnosis?

This previously healthy 21-year-old man presents with recent onset of crampy abdominal pain, tenesmus, and occasionally bloody diarrhea, accompanied by low-grade fever, abdominal tenderness to palpation, guaiac positive stool, and mild anemia. The differential diagnosis includes infective enteritis with *Campylobacter, Salmonella, Shigella, Yersinia, Entamoeba histolytica*, or invasive *E. coli;* antibiotic-associated colitis with *C. difficile*; CMV colitis in an AIDS patient; proctitis due to gonorrhea, chlamydia, HSV, or syphilis; radiation colitis; ischemic colitis in an elderly patient; and inflammatory bowel disease (IBD), a category which includes Crohn's disease and ulcerative colitis.

The patient has not been irradiated and is too young for atherosclerotic ischemic colitis. He could have ischemic colitis due to a mesenteric vasculitis, but has no other vasculitic symptoms. He has not taken any antibiotics in the last 6 months. Stool for bacterial culture, ova, and parasites should be sent. RPR and HIV serologies are also worth considering. A flexible sigmoidoscopy or colonoscopy with biopsies could make the diagnosis of infectious colitis or inflammatory bowel disease. The patient's sexual history makes infectious proctitis less likely, and his travel and food histories, as well as the duration of his symptoms, make infective enteritis unlikely. Inflammatory bowel disease is a concern.

CASE CONTINUED

Over the ensuing week, an RPR and HIV ELISA are negative, as are three stool samples for bacterial pathogens, ova, and parasites, as well as *C. difficile* toxin. You schedule a colonoscopy. The patient's symptoms continue.

QUESTIONS

81. Which of the following are helpful in diagnosing Crohn's disease?
    A. Colonoscopy showing ulcers, skip lesions, or granulomas
    B. Clinical picture of colitis, plus the finding of ulcerations, strictures, or fistulas on upper GI radiography with small bowel follow-through and barium enema
    C. Combined pANCA and ASCA (anti-*Saccharomyces cerevisiae* antibody) testing
    D. All of the above

82. Which of the following are helpful in diagnosing ulcerative colitis?
    A. Colonoscopy or sigmoidoscopy showing ulcerations, friability, and edema beginning in the rectum and extending proximally w/o skip lesions
    B. Upper GI radiography with small bowel follow-through and barium enema
    C. Combined pANCA and ASCA testing
    D. All of the above
    E. (A) and (C)

83. The treatment for Crohn's disease includes all of the following *except*:
    A. 5-Aminosalicylic acid agents
    B. Elective colectomy
    C. Corticosteroids
    D. Azathioprine or mercaptopurine
    E. Anti-TNF antibody

84. The treatment for ulcerative colitis includes all of the following *except*:
    A. 5-Aminosalicylic acid agents
    B. Corticosteroids
    C. Cyclosporine
    D. Elective colectomy
    E. Prophylactic antibiotics

CC/ID: 41-year-old man presents with abdominal pain, nausea and vomiting.

HPI: M.I. was in his usual state of good health until the night before admission, when he was kept awake by a dull periumbilical discomfort, which had progressed to nonradiating, nonpositional pain by the morning. He vomited shortly after trying to drink a cup of tea, and has been unable to take food or liquid by mouth since. He had a small, loose stool on the morning of admission. Because the pain has worsened, he presented to the hospital this afternoon. He denies fevers, shaking chills, and recent weight loss. The remainder of his ROS is also negative, and he denies abdominal trauma.

PMHx: Appendectomy at age 12.　　**Meds:** None　　**All:** NKDA.

SHx: Married, with two children; monogamous. Works as a carpenter. Former cigarette smoker, quit 5 years ago; 2 to 3 beers/week. No recent travel, wilderness exposures.

VS: Temp 38.1°, BP 110/70, HR 100, RR 18; O$_2$ sat 98% on RA

PE: *Gen:* thin, well-developed man in moderate discomfort; alert, awake, conversant. *Neck:* JVP flat; no adenopathy or thyromegaly; 2+ carotids no bruits. *Lungs:* CTA. *CV:* RRR, normal S$_1$S$_2$; no murmurs or rubs. *Abdomen:* Soft, ND; hypoactive BS; periumbilical tenderness to palpation, without rebound; no HSM. *Rectal:* normal tone; smooth NT prostate; no masses; guaiac-positive. *Ext:* no cyanosis, clubbing, edema, rashes, or livedo reticularis; no arthropathy. *Neuro:* nonfocal.

Labs: Na 140; K 4.0; Cl 107; HCO$_3$ 24; BUN 20; Cr 1.1; glucose 75. UA normal. WBC 16,000; Hct 42; Plt 260,000. Transaminases, bilirubin, alkaline phosphatase, amylase all unremarkable. KUB: No infiltrates, cardiomegaly, or subdiaphragmatic free air. Nondistended bowel, with multiple air-fluid levels.

THOUGHT QUESTIONS
- How would you summarize this patient's presentation?
- What could be causing his abdominal pain?
- Do you want to send him home or admit him?

This 41-year-old man presents with 24 hours of worsening periumbilical abdominal pain, vomiting, low-grade fever, minimal stool output, a tender but nonacute-appearing abdominal exam, guaiac-positive stool, and a leukocytosis. KUB shows signs of ileus, but no perforation.

This patient has already undergone appendectomy, which removes a leading cause of periumbilical pain and leukocytosis. The combination of pain, fever, bloody stool (inferred by the guaiac-positive rectal exam), and leukocytosis is concerning for gastroenteritis with an invasive organism or inflammatory bowel disease. However, the lack of diarrhea, as well as evidence of ileus on radiography, points away from these. The symptoms are not particularly consistent with a peptic ulcer, gallbladder disease, or splenic abscess. A partial small bowel obstruction due to occult carcinoma or lymphoma is entirely possible. Finally, periumbilical pain out of proportion to exam findings, accompanied by a leukocytosis is concerning for mesenteric ischemia.

Many patients with suspected gastroenteritis are sent home with antibiotics and instructions to return to the ED should their condition worsen, or should they be unable to tolerate oral intake. Because this patient's diagnosis remains mysterious and could include bowel catastrophe, and because he cannot tolerate PO intake, you decide to admit him for observation and IV fluids.

CASE CONTINUED

You start IV fluids, and send the patient's stool for O+P and bacterial culture. In addition, you plan to perform serial abdominal exams every 3 hours, and consider ordering an abdominal CT scan, starting antibiotics, and asking the GI service to evaluate the patient for colonoscopy. When you check on the patient 3 hours later, his condition appears to have worsened. He is groaning in pain, and does not want to move. His skin is pale and clammy. His temperature is 38.9°C, BP 105/70 after a liter of fluid, HR 110, and RR 20 and shallow. His abdomen is slightly distended, and no longer soft, and it is diffusely tender to light palpation.

QUESTIONS

85. The *least* crucial test(s) at this point would be:
    A. Repeat CBC and chemistry panel, plus type and cross
    B. Abdominal CT
    C. Arterial blood gas
    D. Repeat KUB
    E. All of the above

86. The WBC is now 20,000. The chemistry panel shows Na of 139, Cl of 102, and HCO_3 of 18 with normal glucose. The ABG comes back as pH 7.27, pCO_2 33, pO_2 90. Which of the following terms best describes the acid–base picture?
    A. Metabolic alkalosis
    B. Non-anion gap metabolic acidosis
    C. Anion gap metabolic acidosis
    D. Respiratory acidosis

87. Your next step would be:
    A. Page the GI fellow for emergent colonoscopy.
    B. Add 2 amps of sodium bicarbonate to the IV fluids.
    C. Page the general surgery resident on call.
    D. Page the interventional radiology fellow for emergent angiography.

88. Which of the following diagnoses is most likely?
    A. Toxic megacolon
    B. Pseudomembranous colitis
    C. Ischemic colitis
    D. Infarcted bowel due to acute mesenteric ischemia

CC/ID: 42-year-old man with AIDS presents with pain while eating.

HPI: C.E. was diagnosed with HIV in 1984 with recent CD4 count of 9 cells/mm^3 and viral load >200,000 copies/mL. C.E. had multiple complications of AIDS in the early phases of his illness but had been doing well throughout most of the 1990s on effective antiretroviral medications. However, C.E. has failed most of his recent highly active antiretroviral (HAART) regimens and elected to stop all HIV medications approximately 3 months ago.

C.E. now presents with a 2-week history of painful swallowing. He describes severe pain with swallowing, slightly worse with solids than liquids, but occurring with both. He denies any feeling of obstruction with swallowing, just burning and pain. C.E. has been avoiding food over the past 2 weeks given this severe pain with eating and has been subsisting on small amounts of Ensure supplements and water. He denies any symptoms of heartburn or positional pain. On ROS, he denies any fevers, skin rashes, chills, night sweats, cough, SOB, abdominal pain, nausea, or vomiting. He has had chronic diarrhea over the past 2 years with multiple negative workups.

PMHx: PCP pneumonia 1984 (presenting diagnosis of AIDS). Cutaneous KS throughout late 1980s. *Salmonella* bacteremia 1985. Appendectomy age 21. Rectal herpes.

All: Penicillin (hives)

Meds: TMP/SMX, 1 tablet PO QD (PCP prophylaxis); azithromycin, 1200 mg PO per week (MAC prophylaxis).

SHx: Homosexual; lives with long-term partner; no smoking; no IVDU; minimal alcohol consumption ranging from 1 to 3 drinks of wine per week.

VS: Temp 37.0°C, BP 102/70, HR 120, RR 16; weight 130 lbs, height 5'10"

PE: *Gen:* very cachectic, tired, pale man. *OP:* severe oral thrush; posterior pharynx erythematous. *LAN:* mild anterior cervical lymphadenopathy. *CV:* RRR, S$_1$S$_2$; tachy with 1/VI systolic murmur LLSB; no rubs or gallops. *Lungs:* CTA bilaterally. *Abdomen:* soft; +BS; NT/ND; no HSM. *Rectal:* loose brown stool; trace guaiac-positive.

Labs: WBC 4.00; Hct 36.2; Plt 105; Na 132; K 3.1; HCO$_3$ 34; Cl 110; BUN 30; Cr 0.5

THOUGHT QUESTIONS
- What is this patient's differential diagnosis?
- What is the best way to ascertain the diagnosis?

The differential diagnosis for odynophagia includes various causes of esophagitis in this severely immunosuppressed patient, such as candida, cytomegalovirus (CMV), herpes simplex virus (HSV), mycobacterium avium-intracellulare (MAI), or idiopathic ulceration. Other noninfectious causes include malignancies, such as Kaposi sarcoma and lymphoma, and non-HIV related esophageal disorders, such as reflux disease or pill esophagitis. As candida and HSV esophagitis are both usually observed with CD4 cell counts <200 cells/mm^3, with CMV, idiopathic ulcers and MAI developing with CD4 cell counts <100 cells/mm^3, this patient is at risk for all of the infectious causes of esophagitis in AIDS. The best way to establish the diagnosis is endoscopy with careful examination of the esophageal mucosa and multiple biopsies.

CASE CONTINUED

An endoscopy was performed (Figure 23-1). Biopsy of one of the confluent plaques is shown in Figure 23-2.

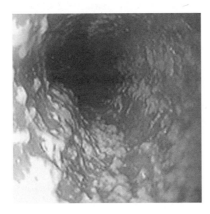

FIGURE 23-1 Esophageal endoscopy showing multiple white plaques and surrounding inflammation on mucosal surface. (Copyrighted material is used with permission of the author, the University of Iowa and Virtual Hospital, www.vh.org.)

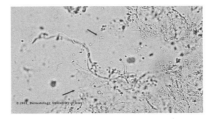

FIGURE 23-2 KOH prep of one of the white plaques seen on endoscopy, showing multiple budding yeast and pseudohyphae. (Copyrighted material is used with permission of the author, the University of Iowa and Virtual Hospital, www.vh.org.)

QUESTIONS

89. The cause of this patient's esophagitis is most likely:
    A. CMV
    B. HSV
    C. KS
    D. *Candida*
    E. HIV idiopathic ulceration

90. Initial treatment for this condition will be:
    A. Amphotericin B
    B. Acyclovir
    C. Fluconazole
    D. Ketoconazole
    E. Ganciclovir

91. What is the usual CD4 count cut-off for initiation of antibiotic prophylaxis for *Pneumocystis*?
    A. CD4 <500 cells/μL
    B. CD4 <250 cells/μL
    C. CD4 <200 cells/μL
    D. CD4 <100 cells/μL
    E. CD4 <50 cells/μL

92. What is the preferred alternative agent to Bactrim for prophylaxis against PCP?
    A. Dapsone
    B. Clindamycin
    C. Primaquine
    D. Trimetrexate
    E. Pyrimethamine

CC/ID: 52-year-old man has sudden onset epigastric pain, nausea, and vomiting.

HPI: A.P. was in his usual state of health until this afternoon, when he experienced the sudden onset of gnawing epigastric pain radiating to his back. The pain was worse when he tried to lie down, and improved when he sat back up. He also reports nausea and vomiting. He denies ripping or tearing pain, chest pain, and SOB. Because his pain did not respond to milk or aspirin, he presented to the ED.

PMHx: Hypertension, hypercholesterolemia

Meds: HCTZ, 25 mg PO QD; simvastatin, 40 mg PO QD   **All:** NKDA.

SHx: 1.5 ppd cigarettes for 20 years; QD EtOH.   **FHx:** Noncontributory.

VS: Temp 39.5°C, BP 150/90 in both arms, HR 110, RR 16

PE: *Gen:* thin man in discomfort, alert and oriented. *HEENT:* PERRLA. OP no lesions. *Neck:* full carotid upstrokes, no bruits, no thyromegaly. Normal JVP. *Lungs:* clear. *CV:* RRR; normal S_1S_2; no murmurs. *Abdomen:* epigastric tenderness to palpation, no rebound or guarding. *Rectal:* guaiac-negative; normal tone.

Labs: WBC 13,000; Hct 39; Plt 250,000; Cr 1.5; normal transaminases, alkaline phosphatase, and bilis; amylase 1100. *CXR:* clear; no subdiaphragmatic free air.

THOUGHT QUESTIONS

- How would you summarize the patient's presentation, and what is the most likely diagnosis?
- If you did not yet know the results of screening labs, what would your differential diagnosis include?

This 52-year-old man, with a history of hypertension, hypercholesterolemia, and alcohol use, presents with the acute onset of positional epigastric pain, nausea and vomiting, fever and tachycardia, a tender upper abdomen, leukocytosis, and an elevated amylase. With this constellation of symptoms and findings, the most likely diagnosis is acute pancreatitis. Neither the clinical presentation nor the serum amylase is entirely specific for acute pancreatitis. Conditions that could present in a similar fashion include aortic dissection or aneurysm, perforated ulcer, small bowel obstruction, acute cholecystitis, or bowel ischemia. The serum amylase can be elevated in small bowel obstruction, after abdominal surgery, or in association with narcotic use (mumps and pregnancy, which can also cause an elevated serum amylase, are unlikely in this case). Sending a serum lipase and obtaining an abdominal CT scan would narrow the diagnosis. Given the patient's systemically ill appearance and fever, two sets of blood cultures are also indicated.

CASE CONTINUED

The lipase is elevated, and the abdominal CT scan with contrast shows an enlarged pancreas, with decreased density in the body and stranding in the surrounding fat (Figure 24). There is no evidence of biliary tract disease.

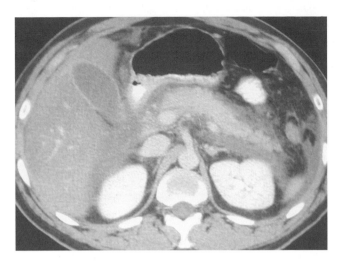

FIGURE 24 Abdominal CT: 52-year-old man with gnawing epigastric pain, nausea, fever, and elevated amylase. (Image provided by Department of Radiology, University of California, San Francisco.)

QUESTIONS

93. All of the additional measurements will be helpful in assessing the severity of the patient's pancreatitis *except*:
    A. Serum LDH on admission
    B. Serial hematocrits in first 48 hours of admission
    C. Serum calcium in first 48 hours of admission
    D. Serial amylase in first 48 hours of admission
    E. BUN and PaO$_2$ in first 48 hours of admission

94. Initial management will include:
    A. NPO, IV fluids and analgesia, NG tube if needed for vomiting
    B. (A) plus cessation of HCTZ
    C. (B) plus ceftriaxone, 1-gram IV q24h
    D. (A) plus endoscopic retrograde cholangiopancreatography (ERCP)

95. Over the next 72 hours, despite appropriate management, the patient becomes sicker. His fever and abdominal pain persist, his WBC rises to 19,000, his BUN rises, and his hematocrit declines by 15%. The initial diagnostic procedure of choice is:
    A. Dynamic helical CT scan of the abdomen with contrast
    B. ERCP
    C. Abdominal ultrasound
    D. Exploratory laparotomy

96. The medical management of necrotizing pancreatitis includes all of the following *except*:
    A. Aggressive supportive care
    B. IV imipenem
    C. Continuous percutaneous drainage alone
    D. CT-guided diagnostic fine-needle aspiration for failure to improve

CASE 25 / TOO MUCH TYLENOL

CC/ID: 32-year-old woman with h/o depression brought to ER in coma.

HPI: L.F. is a 32-year-old woman generally in good health except for a long history of depression. She had been doing well until 3 months ago when she suffered a relationship breakup with her long-time boyfriend. Since then, per friends, she had been having trouble sleeping and eating and has frequent bouts of crying. She was recently fired for failure to appear at work for a week. L.F.'s brother entered her apartment on the day of admission after her friends had tried to call her repeatedly for 3 days and found her lying on the floor, unresponsive in a pool of vomit. Lying next to her were two empty bottles of Tylenol and a note reading, "I am sorry, but I can't live without him." An ambulance was called. The patient was nasally intubated in the field and brought to the ER.

PMHx: Depression, no prior suicide attempts.   **Meds:** Zoloft, 150 mg PO QD   **All:** NKDA

SHx: No h/o smoking; rare EtOH; no IVDU or drugs; lives alone; dental hygienist.

VS: Temp 38.0°C, BP 85/50, HR 115, RR 18, O_2 sat 100% on FIO_2 of 1.0

PE: *Gen:* nonresponsive, jaundiced, intubated woman lying in gurney. *HEENT:* PERRLA; severe bleeding around nasal intubation site; sclera icteric; OP clear. *Neck/CV/Lungs:* WNL. *Abdomen:* hypoactive BS; liver edge palpable 4 cm below RCM; no splenomegaly. *Ext:* no edema. *Rectal:* brown stool; heme positive. *Skin:* no palmar erythema; no spider angiomata; no petechial rashes. *Neuro:* unresponsive except to deep painful stimuli; face symmetric; DTRs 1+ ankles, knees; Babinski's equivocal.

Labs: WBC 3.2; Hct 30.2; Plts 46,000. Na 133; K 4.5; Cl 112; HCO_3 16; BUN 90; Cr 4.6; Glu 43; Total bili 24.6 (direct 21.0); AST 14,300; ALT 5400; Alk phos 420; Alb 2.9; PT 45.5; INR 5.8; PTT >100; ABG in the field was 7.27/50/50; Serum β-HCG negative; hepatitis A IgM and IgG negative; HepBeAb negative; HepBeAg negative; HepBcore Ab negative; HepBsAb negative; HepBsAg negative; HepC Ab negative; ceruloplasmin negative; ANA negative; acetaminophen level 210 μg/mL. *ECG:* sinus tachycardia, otherwise WNL. *CXR:* clear.

THOUGHT QUESTIONS

- What are the clinical stages of acetaminophen poisoning?
- How is the prognosis and need for treatment of acetaminophen overdose assessed?
- What are the criteria for orthotopic liver transplantation in patients with acute liver failure due to acetaminophen poisoning?

The clinical presentation of acetaminophen poisoning is usually divided into four stages:

Stage 1 (12 to 24 hours after ingestion): Nausea, vomiting, diaphoresis, and anorexia may be present and lab tests are usually normal.

Stage 2 (24 to 72 hours after ingestion): Symptoms may have decreased, although tenderness in the RUQ may be present. ALT, AST, and Alk phos levels are usually elevated; PT may be prolonged.

Stage 3 (72 to 96 hours after ingestion): Fulminant hepatic failure with various manifestations of hepatic encephalopathy, coagulopathy, respiratory failure, renal failure, jaundice. Severe lab abnormalities, including massive elevations in AST/ALT and coagulation parameters, as well as profound hypoglycemia. Death from hepatic failure can occur in this stage.

Stage 4 (7 to 8 days after ingestion): Hepatic recovery in those who survive stage 3.

Serum acetaminophen (APAP) concentrations are used to predict prognosis and need for antidote therapy. Based on prognostic correlations obtained from data in adults, the Rumack-Matthew nomogram (Figure 25) plots serum APAP concentrations in relation to time since ingestion to determine a "treatment line." If the serum APAP value falls above the line of the nomogram upon adjustment for time, patients are at high risk of liver injury and protective therapy is indicated.

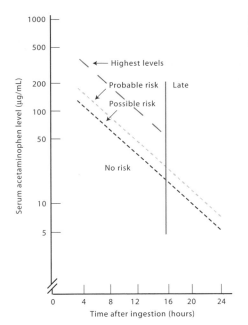

FIGURE 25 Rumack-Matthew nomogram showing serum acetaminophen concentrations in relation to time since ingestion. (Illustration by Shawn Girsberger Graphic Design.)

Note that an APAP level of 50 μg/mL may pose no risk of hepatocellular injury 4 hours after ingestion, but poses a significant risk of liver damage >16 hours after ingestion. In terms of criteria for orthotopic liver transplantation in patients with acute liver failure secondary to acetaminophen poisoning, the biochemical criteria established are pH <7.3 or INR >5.5 and serum creatinine >3.4 mg/dL.

CASE CONTINUED

L.F. was in fulminant hepatic failure and was taken to the ICU for intensive monitoring and management. She was immediately placed on the liver transplant list, class I. Nasal intubation was replaced with endotracheal intubation, with pre-infusion of fresh frozen plasma in the face of traumatic bleeding. Given that this patient had APAP levels >200 μg/mL probably 48 to 72 hours after ingestion, protective therapy for acetaminophen poisoning was administered. Patient was also started on intravenous dextrose. Vitamin K was administered intravenously for the coagulopathy. Head CT showed cerebral edema and mannitol was initiated. Approximately 12 hours after admission, a liver donor was located. As the patient was being prepared for surgery, her cardiac tracing became asystolic. Despite vigorous efforts to revive her, the patient expired.

QUESTIONS

97. What is the antidote or protective treatment for acetaminophen poisoning called?
    A. Bicarbonate
    B. *N*-acetylcysteine (NAC)
    C. Charcoal
    D. S-adenosyl methionine
    E. Salicylates

98. Which of the following coagulation factors made by the liver are *not* vitamin K dependent?
    A. Factor II
    B. Factor V
    C. Factor VII
    D. Factor IX
    E. Factor X

99. Ceruloplasmin is a test performed for the diagnosis of which condition (that can lead to liver failure)?
    A. Hematochromatosis
    B. Glycogen storage disease
    C. Reye syndrome
    D. Budd-Chiari syndrome
    E. Wilson's disease

100. Which of the following hepatitis viruses is the *least* likely to cause fulminant hepatic failure as its initial presentation?
    A. Hepatitis A
    B. Hepatitis B
    C. Hepatitis C
    D. Hepatitis D superinfecting hepatitis B carrier
    E. Hepatitis E

CC/ID: 47-year-old man with fever, increasing abdominal girth, yellow skin, and drowsiness.

HPI: S.P. has a history of chronic hepatitis C virus infection complicated by cirrhosis, portal hypertension, and ascites. The latter is controlled with furosemide and spironolactone. Roughly 10 days ago he began to gain weight and to notice a persistent increase in his abdominal girth, despite continuing to take his diuretics. Last night, he complained of abdominal discomfort. This morning, he was difficult to arouse and appeared disoriented. His wife brought him to the hospital. When you try to interview the patient, he is too confused to give a reliable history. His wife denies that he has complained of chills or sweats, headache, chest pain, cough, joint swelling, or rash. He has had one firm, nonbloody, non-tarry bowel movement in the last 2 days. He has had no hematemesis.

PMHx: Chronic HCV infection diagnosed 10 years ago. No history of varices. CT negative for liver masses 6 months ago. On liver transplant list.

Meds: Furosemide, 160 mg PO QD; spironolactone, 400 mg PO QD; low-sodium diet   **All:** NKDA

SHx: Quit IV heroin 15 years ago; quit EtOH 7 years ago. Married, two teenage children.

VS: Temp 39°C, BP 110/60, HR 100, RR 18

PE: *Gen:* icteric man, sleepy but arousable. *HEENT:* icteric sclerae, palate, frenulum. *Lungs/Chest:* clear bilaterally, with gynecomastia. *CV:* tachy, regular, normal S_1S_2. *Abdomen:* protuberant, with bulging flanks and fluid wave; can't assess HSM; spider nevi on chest, abdominal wall; dilated superficial veins; abdomen diffusely tender to palpation. *GU:* testicular atrophy. *Rectal:* guaiac negative. *Ext:* peripheral wasting, palmar erythema, asterixis. *Neuro:* uncooperative with exam; alert to person.

Labs: Na^+ 129; K^+ 3; Cr 1.8; Alb 1.5; Total bili 4.0; Direct bili 3.0; INR 1.8; WBC 13,000; Hct 39; Plt 50,000; Urine Na^+ <10 mEq/L. KUB: clear chest; no intra-abdominal free air, dilated bowel loops or air-fluid levels.

THOUGHT QUESTIONS
- How would you summarize this patient's presentation?
- What is your most likely unifying diagnosis?

This 47-year-old man with end-stage, cirrhotic liver disease presents with ascites unresponsive to diuretics for the last 10 days, and now fever, abdominal pain, jaundice, and confusion. The most commonly encountered complications of cirrhosis, regardless of the cause, are portal hypertension with ascites; coagulopathy; bleeding from esophageal or gastric varices; hepatic encephalopathy; spontaneous bacterial peritonitis; hepatocellular carcinoma; the hepatorenal syndrome; and ultimately death from liver failure. This patient demonstrates several of these processes. First, his ascites has become refractory to standard combination therapy with furosemide and spironolactone. Second, the presence of confusion, stupor, and asterixis strongly suggest hepatic encephalopathy, which occurs when the failing liver can no longer metabolize neurotoxins originating in the gut. Some of the common conditions predisposing to hepatic encephalopathy include infection, gastrointestinal bleeding, narcotic and sedative use, and volume deficiency. Third, the constellation of fever, ascites, and abdominal pain is very suggestive for spontaneous bacterial peritonitis (SBP), an intra-abdominal infection which is lethal if not promptly diagnosed and treated. SBP probably results from seeding of ascitic fluid during transient episodes of bacteremia, and should be ruled out by performing diagnostic paracentesis in any patient with ascites and abdominal pain. While the combination of fever and altered mental status is always concerning for meningitis, the most likely explanation for this patient's presentation is that his ascites, now unresponsive to diuretics, has become infected, leading to SBP and, in turn, hepatic encephalopathy.

CASE CONTINUED

Diagnostic paracentesis yields 10 cc of cloudy, yellow fluid. You draw two sets of peripheral blood cultures, start intravenous antibiotics, and consider how to address the patient's encephalopathy and massive ascites.

QUESTIONS

101. When analyzing the patient's ascites, it is important to determine all of the following *except*:
    A. Albumin
    B. Glucose
    C. Cell count and differential
    D. Culture

102. Appropriate empiric antibiotics for SBP could consist of:
    A. Gentamicin plus Metronidazole.
    B. Cefotaxime ± Ampicillin.
    C. Ampicillin/Sulbactam or Ticarcillin/Clavulanate or Piperacillin/Tazobactam.
    D. (B) or (C).

103. Appropriate therapy for hepatic encephalopathy could include any of the following *except*:
    A. Neomycin, 0.5–1.0 gram PO q6–12h
    B. Lactulose PO or by retention enema
    C. Lactulose plus neomycin
    D. Nothing. The encephalopathy will resolve once the underlying hepatic decompensation is reversed. Agitation can be managed with diazepam.

104. To relieve the patient of his massive ascites, you perform a large volume paracentesis, drawing off 8 liters of fluid. Two days later, you note that his abdominal girth is increasing again. Therapeutic options could include all of the following *except*:
    A. Periodic large-volume paracenteses
    B. Placement of a transjugular intrahepatic portosystemic shunt (TIPS)
    C. Placement of a percutaneous drain
    D. Liver transplantation

CC/ID: 50-year-old woman with fever, abdominal pain, and foot drop.

HPI: P.N. was in her usual state of health until 6 weeks ago, when she noted the onset of fatigue and malaise, which she ascribed to early menopause. She then developed myalgias in her limbs, and an occasional headache. In the past 2 weeks, she has been experiencing diffuse, postprandial abdominal pain, sometimes with nausea. Yesterday evening she developed a left foot drop and decided to come to the ED. She denies chills, drenching night sweats, stiff neck, sinus congestion, cough, SOB, chest pain, diarrhea, or rash. She has felt "feverish."

PMHx: Cholecystectomy at age 35. G2P2. Seasonal allergies.

Meds: Antihistamines as needed   **All:** Penicillin (rash)

SHx: Divorced book editor. Non-smoker; occasional EtOH; no IVDU. Denies animal/tick contact.

FHx: Older sister has breast cancer; father died of colon cancer at age 70.

VS: Temp 100.5°F, BP 150/95, HR 90, RR 12, O$_2$ sat 99% on RA

PE: *Gen:* thin woman in no distress, who appears chronically ill. *HEENT:* normal eye exam; no mucosal ulcerations or sinus tenderness. *Neck:* supple, no adenopathy or thyromegaly. *Lungs/Chest:* clear. No breast masses. *CV:* RRR, normal S$_1$S$_2$, no murmurs, rubs, heaves. *Abdomen:* soft, NT, no RUQ tenderness. No masses, no organomegaly. *Rectal:* no masses, trace heme positive. Normal tone. *Ext:* livedo reticularis on bilateral lower extremities. No arthropathy. 2+ peripheral pulses bilaterally in all four extremities. *Neuro:* absent dorsiflexion on left foot; otherwise normal.

Labs: WBC 13, Hct 34, Cr 1.1, UA normal. *CXR:* normal.

THOUGHT QUESTIONS
- What broad categories would you include in this patient's differential diagnosis?
- What tests would you order to help narrow your diagnosis?

This middle-aged woman presents with a progressive, multisystem illness of 1 to 2 months' duration, consisting of constitutional symptoms, myalgias, headache, postprandial abdominal pain, and now a peripheral mononeuropathy. In addition, she presents with a low-grade fever, elevated blood pressure, mild leukocytosis, and mild anemia.

The subacute, progressive, constitutional nature of this syndrome, while nonspecific, suggests an infection, malignancy, or inflammatory disorder. Possible infections include infective endocarditis, splenic or hepatic abscess, and HIV disease. The lack of contact with ticks or animals rules out zoonotic infections, while the lack of pulmonary findings in this ostensibly immunocompetent patient makes tuberculosis unlikely. Cancers of the GI, GU, and gynecologic tract are possible, as is mesenteric or retroperitoneal lymphoma. Leukemia, while possible, is less likely in the setting of a normal peripheral smear.

The constellation of peripheral mononeuropathy, chronic, progressive constitutional symptoms, and abdominal pain is suspicious for a systemic vasculitis. These disorders are characterized by an inflammatory necrosis of blood vessels, and can be primary processes (for example, polyarteritis nodosa [PAN]/microscopic polyangiitis; Wegener's granulomatosis; giant cell arteritis; and Takayasu's arteritis) or be associated with underlying autoimmune diseases (such as lupus or viral hepatitis with cryoglobulinemia). When approaching a patient with a systemic illness of unclear cause, it is important to keep the vasculitic syndromes in mind, as they can be highly destructive, lethal, and difficult to diagnose. In addition to the labs reported above, two sets of blood cultures and urine culture should be sent, as well as serologic tests that might help diagnose a specific vasculitis. These include ANA, cANCA, pANCA, HBV, and HCV, as well as HCV RNA and cryoglobulins. An abdominal CT scan would screen for fluid collections and masses.

QUESTIONS

105. Blood and urine cultures are negative. The pANCA titer is positive. The abdominal CT scan is normal. The most likely diagnosis is:
    A. Infective endocarditis
    B. PAN
    C. Lymphoma
    D. Wegener's granulomatosis
    E. Lupus

106. This disease is *least* likely to involve the:
    A. Brain
    B. Kidney
    C. Skin
    D. Lung

107. Further workup should include:
    A. Nerve biopsy in the affected leg
    B. Aortic and mesenteric angiography
    C. Open lung biopsy
    D. Magnetic resonance angiography of the brain

108. In treating this patient, you should consider all of the following *except*:
    A. Steroids
    B. Cyclophosphamide
    C. Radiation
    D. Consultation with a rheumatologist

CC/ID: 19-year-old woman has fatigue and SOB, stating, "I feel like I'm gonna die."

HPI: Except for mild dysuria, D.K., a 19-year-old woman, was in her usual good state of health until 2 days before admission, when she began to experience constant thirst and a marked increase in urinary frequency. She became progressively fatigued and felt "slow." This morning, she felt short of breath, exhausted, and dizzy, "as if I were drunk." Her stomach began to hurt, and she became nauseated, vomiting several times. She asked a friend to drive her to the hospital because she thought she was going to die. She reports a mild headache in the last half-day, but no neck pain or stiffness. She denies chills, cough, diarrhea, or vaginal discharge. She is not currently sexually active with a partner.

PMHx: 2 to 3 UTIs in the past year. No surgeries. Normal menstrual periods.   **Meds:** None

All: NKDA   **SHx:** Student. No cigarettes; occasional social EtOH; no illicit substances.

VS: Temp 36.5°C, BP 98/60, HR 110, RR 24, O_2 sat 99% on RA

PE: *Gen:* thin woman breathing deeply and quickly, with sunken cheeks. *HEENT:* PERRLA; dry OP. Unpleasantly fruity-smelling breath. *Neck:* supple; no thyromegaly; flat JVP. *Lungs:* clear bilaterally, with equal breath sounds. *CV:* tachycardic, regular, normal S_1S_2; flow murmur. *Abdomen:* soft, with mild epigastric tenderness to palpation; no guarding. *Ext:* no clubbing, cyanosis, or edema. *Skin:* skin tenting on forehead, forearms. No rashes. *Neuro:* oriented to person, place, date.

Labs: Na 145; K^+ 5.5; Cl^- 107; HCO_3 13; BUN 40; Cr 1.5; Glucose 600; WBC 13,000; Hct 42; Plt 350,000; Serum ketones + 1:32; UA with 4+ ketones, +leukocyte esterase, +nitrate. ABG: 7.20/26/95/14 on RA. *CXR:* clear.

THOUGHT QUESTIONS
- How would you classify the patient's acid–base status using the ABG and serum electrolytes?
- Summarize her presentation using the history, physical examination, and lab work, including acid–base status.
- What is the most likely diagnosis?

The pH of 7.20 indicates an acidosis, and the low serum bicarbonate and low pCO_2 confirm that it is primarily metabolic, rather than respiratory. The anion gap (Na − (Cl + HCO_3)) of 25 is (much) greater than normal (12), indicating an anion gap metabolic acidosis. Finally, you can use Winter's formula to see whether the patient is compensating for her underlying metabolic acidosis by increasing her respiratory CO_2 excretion; if the $pCO_2 = 1.5 \times$ (serum HCO_3) + 8 ± 2, then there is a metabolic acidosis with respiratory compensation. The list of conditions and toxicities that present with a positive anion-gap metabolic acidosis is given by the acronym MUDPILES (*M*ethanol, *U*remia, *D*iabetic and alcoholic ketoacidosis, *P*araldehyde, *I*NH and iron, *L*actic acidosis, *E*thylene glycol, *S*alicylates). With a history of polyuria and polydipsia, an exam notable for dehydration and Kussmaul respirations, and labs showing hyperglycemia, elevated serum ketones, and an anion gap metabolic acidosis, the patient presents with the classic picture of diabetic ketoacidosis (DKA). The pathophysiology of DKA involves the lack of insulin production, with concomitant glucagon release. This leads to gluconeogenesis, hyperglycemia, and lipolysis, which in turn produce an osmotic diuresis and dehydration, and the conversion of mobilized fat stores into ketoacids. The goal of treatment is to correct the dehydration with fluids and reverse the ketoacidosis with insulin, while carefully monitoring and correcting the related electrolyte disturbances. DKA can be the first announcement that a patient has type I diabetes mellitus, or can occur in a patient already known to have the disease. DKA occasionally affects patients thought to have type II disease as well.

CASE CONTINUED

While you were figuring out the patient's acid–base status and trying to remember Winter's formula, the nurse has started an IV line and is wondering aloud whether you plan to treat the patient in this world or the next.

QUESTIONS

109. Immediate therapy for DKA includes all of the following *except*:
    A. IV fluids
    B. Regular insulin, "IV push," as a loading dose, plus a regular insulin drip
    C. NPH insulin
    D. Setting up a flow chart to monitor the patient's response to therapy

110. Concerned about the elevated potassium of 5.5, you decide to:
    A. Lower the potassium with Kayexalate.
    B. Lower the potassium with extra insulin and albuterol.
    C. Do nothing.
    D. Give potassium once you have started treating the patient's DKA.

111. One hour after starting treatment, the patient's blood glucose is still 600. You decide to:
    A. Wait for the insulin drip to start working
    B. Increase the rate of the insulin drip
    C. Repeat the loading dose of insulin
    D. Give bicarbonate IV

112. To look for a medical event that might have incited this episode of DKA, you order or perform any of the following *except*:
    A. Chest x-ray
    B. Urine microscopy and culture
    C. Blood cultures
    D. Chest and abdominal CT
    E. Pelvic exam with cultures

CC/ID: 38-year-old woman presents with fatigue and depression.

HPI: L.T. presents to her primary care physician with complaints of a general feeling of fatigue and "mental slowness." She was formerly in good health, but feels that her fatigue has been increasing over the past year, accompanied by depression with sadness, frequent crying episodes, difficulty sleeping, difficulty concentrating, and poor memory. She reports a weight gain of around 10 lbs. in the past year, despite no increase in food intake. She denies any fever but feels that she "is always cold, even when it's warm outside"; denies night sweats, cough, SOB, abdominal pain, nausea, vomiting, or urinary symptoms. She admits to increasing constipation, with BM occurring every 2 to 3 days at times, but no blood or mucus in stool. Her menstrual periods have been irregular, occurring every 21 to 35 days, and she feels that bleeding is heavier than usual during her menses. LMP was 1 week ago and L.T. is not currently sexually active. She has no unusual vaginal discharge or lesions. She denies any rashes but feels that skin is drier than usual and complains of thinning, brittle hair. She denies joint abnormalities.

PMHx: Uterine fibroids

Meds: Recently started taking St. John's wort over-the-counter for depression   **All:** NKDA

SHx: No h/o current smoking although smoked 10 years ago (1 ppd for 5 years); drinks 1 glass of wine every night; occasional marijuana use but no other illicit drugs or IV drug use. Patient is a family care physician; currently single since breakup with long-term boyfriend 6 months ago; not sexually active at this time.

FHx: No h/o cancer, depression, autoimmune, or endocrine disorders in family.

VS: Afebrile, BP 128/78, HR 58, RR 12, O_2 sat 96% on RA

PE: *Gen:* depressed-appearing pale female in NAD. *HEENT:* thin coarse hair; OP clear with mildly dry mucus membranes. *Neck:* nontender, diffusely enlarged thyroid gland; no nodules appreciated; no LAN or JVD. *CV:* RRR S_1S_2; no murmurs, gallops, or rubs. *Lungs:* CTA bilaterally. *Abdomen:* soft; hypoactive BS; NT/ND; no HSM. *Ext:* no edema present. *Skin:* dry and coarse; no rashes. *Neuro:* intact except for mildly delayed deep tendon reflexes; strength 5/5 throughout; normal Mini-Mental Status Examination except for difficulty with recall of 3 objects at the 5-minute time point (2/3).

Labs: WBC 6.50 with normal differential; Hct 35.0 with MCV 100; Plt 180,000; Na 132; K 3.5; BUN 10; Cr 0.5; glu 95; Free T_4 4 µg/dL; TSH 12 µg/dL

THOUGHT QUESTIONS

- What are the most likely causes of this patient's condition?
- What is the pathophysiology of this condition?
- What further diagnostic tests would be helpful in specifying the cause?

This patient has a diagnosis of hypothyroidism per her symptoms, physical examination, and laboratory evaluation. The prevalence of hypothyroidism increases with age and is more commonly observed in women than men. The basic mechanisms of hypothyroidism can be divided into those that impair thyroid function (primary hypothyroidism) and those that principally involve hypothalamic-pituitary function (secondary hypothyroidism). In primary disease, the hypothalamus responds with an increased output of thyrotropin-releasing hormone (TRH), which triggers pituitary thyrotropin (TSH) secretion. This in turn stimulates thyroid gland enlargement, goiter formation, and the preferential synthesis of triiodothyronine (T_3) over thyroxine (T_4). In secondary hypothyroidism, the TSH response is inadequate, the gland is normal or reduced in size, and T_4 synthesis and T_3 synthesis are equally reduced. The most common form of primary hypothyroidism is Hashimoto thyroiditis, which results from autoimmune antibody production, resulting in blockade of thyroid TSH receptors, impairment of thyroxine production, or inhibition of thyroxine release: TSH receptors and microsomal enzymes (e.g., peroxidase) are among the targeted antigens. Early Hashimoto thyroiditis is usually manifested by a diffusely enlarged nontender gland; late Hashimoto's usually results in a small, rubbery, nontender goiter. Laboratory markers present in this condition include antithyroglobulin antibodies and antithyroid peroxidase (or antimicrosomal) antibodies. Secondary hypothyroidism occurs most commonly as a result of injury to thyrotropes by a functioning or non-functioning pituitary adenoma. Many other forms of sellar or suprasellar disease can produce the same net result, which is inadequate production of TSH leading to an atrophic thyroid gland and hypothyroidism.

CASE CONTINUED

Antithyroglobulin and antimicrosomal antibody tests were both positive and L.T. was given a diagnosis of hypothyroidism secondary to Hashimoto thyroiditis. Therapy was initiated with levothyroxine.

QUESTIONS

113. Which of the following serum concentrations are increased in primary hypothyroidism?
    A. Sodium
    B. Hematocrit
    C. Cholesterol
    D. Calcium
    E. Free T_4 index

114. Which of the following is *not* a cause of primary hypothyroidism?
    A. Subtotal thyroidectomy
    B. Iodide deficiency
    C. Postirradiation disease
    D. Postpartum thyroiditis
    E. Pituitary macroadenoma

115. A tender, enlarged, asymmetric thyroid gland with transient glandular dysfunction is primarily seen in the following disorder:
    A. Postirradiation disease
    B. Subacute thyroiditis
    C. Postpartum thyroiditis
    D. Hashimoto thyroiditis
    E. Infiltration of the gland secondary to amyloidosis

116. Subacute thyroiditis usually follows which clinical syndrome?
    A. Pregnancy
    B. Cancer of the thymus
    C. Viral upper respiratory infection
    D. Iodide deficiency
    E. Autoimmune disorder

CC/ID: 62-year-old woman is brought to the ER with confusion.

HPI: H.C. was brought into the ER by ambulance with disorientation and somnolence. She was in good health until approximately 2 months ago when she started complaining to her daughter about general fatigue, worsening constipation, occasional night sweats, diffuse body aches, anorexia, and general irritability. She felt her symptoms were secondary to depression after the death of her husband 8 months earlier and refused to seek medical care, stating that "they would just tell me to get my head shrunk." Her daughter notes that her mother has lost about 15 lbs. in the past 4 months, seemed to be urinating very frequently, and was generally lethargic and withdrawn. No apparent fevers, chills, cough, SOB, abdominal pain, diarrhea, or burning with urination. Daughter went to see her mother today after a lapse of 3 days and found her lying on the floor in her nightgown with her eyes closed. H.C. was difficult to arouse but was able to open her eyes after heavy shaking and say her daughter's name. Her daughter called 911.

PMHx: Hypertension

Meds: Lisinopril, 20 mg PO QD (with variable compliance; patient rarely sought health care)

All: Sulfa drugs (rash)

SHx: No h/o smoking; minimal EtOH intake; no illicit drugs. Homemaker; recently widowed and now lives alone; has one daughter (nearby) and a son who lives in England.

VS: Temp 36.0; BP 115/70; HR 108; RR 16

PE: *Gen:* rather frail woman looking older than her stated age, lying in the gurney with her eyes closed, occasionally moaning. *Neuro:* somnolent and arousable only with vigorous stimulation. Oriented to name but not to place or date and couldn't answer any other questions. PERRLA; tongue midline, tone normal and symmetric, sensation grossly intact and DTRs 1+ throughout. *HEENT:* mucus membranes dry; whitish-gray plaque-like depositions across the surface of her corneas arrayed in a band-like pattern. *Neck:* ~1 cm left-sided supraclavicular nodes *CV:* RRR S_1S_2; tachy; no murmurs, gallops, or rubs. *Breasts:* normal contour; approximately 2×2 cm firm mass on left breast at 3 o'clock position; left-sided axillary LAN ~1 cm. *Lungs:* CTA bilaterally. *Abdomen:* +BS; soft; patient groaned with palpation in RUQ region; liver enlarged to ~9 cm; no splenomegaly. *Skin:* reduced capillary refill and skin tenting present; scattered ecchymoses over all extremities.

Labs: WBC 6.50; Hgb 10.3; Plt 300K; Na 147; K 3.7; Cl 115; HCO_3 29; BUN 23; Cr 1.4; Ca 14.8; Phos 1.9; LFTs WNL except for albumin of 3.0. *CXR:* Figure 30-1. *Abdominal CT:* Figure 30-2.

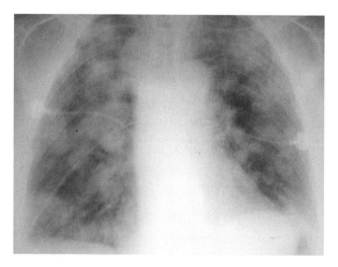

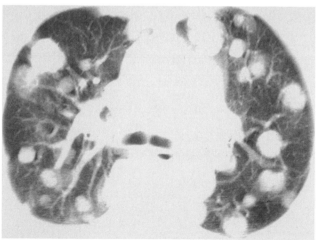

FIGURE 30-1 CXR showing multiple nodules throughout bilateral lung fields. (Image provided by Department of Radiology, University of California, San Francisco.)

FIGURE 30-2 Abdominal CT scan showing multiple low-density lesions throughout the liver. (Image provided by Department of Radiology, University of California, San Francisco.)

THOUGHT QUESTIONS
- What is the differential diagnosis of hypercalcemia?
- What is the most likely cause of H.C.'s hypercalcemia?
- What is the cause of the ocular finding depicted above?

TABLE 30. Causes of Hypercalcemia

Parathyroid related: Parathyroid adenoma; sporadic, familial (multiple endocrine neoplasia types I and II); parathyroid carcinoma

Malignancy related: Tumor metastases to bone; humoral hypercalcemia of malignancy

Vitamin-D related: Vitamin D intoxication; excessive production of vitamin D in granulomatous disorders (e.g., TB, sarcoidosis)

Associated with high bone turnover: Thyrotoxicosis hypoadrenalism; immobilization with increased bone turnover (e.g., Paget)

Drug related: Thiazide diuretics, lithium, theophylline toxicity, estrogens, and antiestrogens

Associated with renal failure: Acute renal failure with rhabdomyolysis; secondary hyperparathyroidism in chronic renal failure; aluminum toxicity

Ingestions: Excessive calcium carbonate ingestion (milk alkali syndrome); vitamin A toxicity

Other: Familial hypocalciuric hypercalcemia

In this case, given the breast mass and the evidence of metastases to both liver and lung, the most likely cause of this patient's hypercalcemia is "humoral hypercalcemia of malignancy." The ocular finding above is called "band keratopathy" and results from the deposition of calcium in the superficial layers of the cornea, usually as a horizontal band starting peripherally and moving centrally. It is associated with hypercalcemia, chronic inflammatory eye conditions, such as uveitis, and topical calcium-containing ocular preparations.

CASE CONTINUED

H.C. became progressively more obtunded in the ED and was admitted to the ICU for intensive monitoring and vigorous fluid replacement. Pamidronate and calcitonin were administered to lower the serum calcium. Within 24 hours, H.C.'s mental status had cleared dramatically with a reduction in her calcium level to 11.9 mg/dL. Given her widely metastatic breast cancer, the patient elected for home comfort care and was discharged on pain medications, with arrangements for periodic pamidronate infusions. She died at her daughter's home 4 weeks later.

QUESTIONS

117. What is the most common cause of hypercalcemia in the outpatient setting?
    A. Malignancy
    B. Dehydration
    C. Thiazide diuretics
    D. Parathyroid adenoma
    E. Vitamin D toxicity

118. Which of the following mechanisms has been most frequently implicated in malignancy-associated hypercalcemia?
    A. Secretion by the tumor of a parathyroid-hormone related peptide
    B. Secretion by the tumor of authentic parathyroid hormone
    C. Secretion by the tumor of 1,25-dihydroxyvitamin D
    D. Tumor metastases to bone with osteolytic activity
    E. Mutations in the extracellular calcium-sensing receptor gene

119. Which malignancy below is *not* typically associated with hypercalcemia?
    A. Breast cancer
    B. Lung cancer
    C. Multiple myeloma
    D. Renal cell carcinoma
    E. Acute myelogenous leukemia

120. The ECG finding most associated with hypercalcemia is the following:
    A. ST segment depressions
    B. Tall peaked T waves
    C. Shortened QT interval
    D. U waves
    E. Flat P waves

CC/ID: 58-year-old Mexican woman brought to the ER with nausea and weakness.

HPI: 58-year-old Mexican woman with long h/o asthma, formerly treated in Mexico. A.I. had multiple hospitalizations 5 years ago for asthma exacerbations with several intubation episodes, but has been doing much better on an OTC medication suggested by her physician in Mexico. She has been on this medication for 5 years and has not needed hospitalization since. A.I. recently immigrated to the U.S. to be with her daughters and ran out of this asthma medication about 3 weeks ago. Since then, A.I. has been feeling mildly SOB, with episodes of wheezing and coughing. Over the past week, she has been feeling weak, tired, and listless, with reduced appetite and complaints of light-headedness when standing up from a sitting position. Over the past few days, she has developed nausea with occasional episodes of vomiting, abdominal cramping, loose brown BM two to three times a day without blood or mucus, arthralgias, and myalgias. She denies any fevers, chills, or urinary symptoms.

PMHx: Long h/o asthma as described above. Mild depression for the past 3 years. Hypertension.

Meds: OTC oral asthma medication and prescribed antihypertensive from Mexico for past 5 years (daughter sent home to obtain medication packages)

All: Penicillin ("can't remember reaction")

SHx: Smokes 1 pack per week for past 30 years; no EtOH or drugs. Widowed and has 5 children; currently living with two daughters in the U.S.

VS: Temp 37.0°C, BP 74/40, HR 105, RR 18, O_2 sat 94% RA (refused orthostatics)

PE: *Gen:* obese woman, lying back in gurney, tremulous and complaining of dizziness *HEENT:* moon facies, OP clear. *Neck:* fat deposition in neck; no thyromegaly or nodules. *Trunk:* central obesity with extremity wasting; fat pad deposition ("buffalo hump") in posterior neck; purple striae over trunk and abdomen with diffuse fine body hair growth. *CV:* RRR S_1S_2; no murmurs, gallops, or rubs. *Lungs:* Mild–moderate end expiratory wheezing but good air movement. *Abdomen:* soft; obese; diffuse abdominal tenderness to palpation without rebound or guarding; ND; no HSM. *Ext:* scattered ecchymoses over LE bilaterally.

Labs: Na 127; K 5.8; Cl 115; HCO_3 22; BUN 40; Cr 0.8; Glu 68; Ca 10.2; Mg 2.0; CBC, TSH, UA and LFTs WNL; Blood cultures × 2 negative. *CXR:* clear.

THOUGHT QUESTIONS
- What diagnosis does the body habitus in this patient suggest?
- What diagnosis do the clinical picture, vital signs, and laboratory values suggest?
- Suggest one unifying diagnosis to this case.

The description of the physical findings in this patient suggests the diagnosis of Cushing's syndrome, a disease that results from prolonged exposure to excess levels of glucocorticoids. Excess cortisol leads to catabolic effects in most tissues, with muscle wasting and weakness peripherally, accompanied by fat deposition centrally in the face, neck, and trunk. Typical Cushing features thus include centripetal obesity, moon facies, and a buffalo hump (fat deposition in the upper back). In the face of cortisol excess, collagen production is impaired, leading to spontaneous ecchymoses, pigmented striae, and poor wound healing; diffuse fine body hair growth, known as lanugo hair, is often observed. Catabolic effects on bone are also seen, leading to increased bone reabsorption, hypercalcemia, and osteoporosis. In the face of continued glucocorticoid exposure, hyperglycemia and impaired cell-mediated immunity are also observed, leading to increased susceptibility to bacterial and fungal pathogens. Hypertension, accelerated atherosclerosis, and psychiatric symptoms, such as psychosis and depression, are common. Syndromes unique to *exogenous* glucocorticoid exposure are aseptic necrosis of the femoral or humeral heads, glaucoma, cataracts, benign intracranial hypertension, and pancreatitis.

The hypotension, hyponatremia, hyperkalemia, hypoglycemia, hypercalcemia, azotemia, and symptomatology of this patient all suggest adrenal insufficiency, and indeed, impending adrenal crisis. One way to unify the diagnosis of physical findings of Cushing's syndrome with a clinical presentation of adrenal crisis in this patient is to postulate the exogenous administration of glucocorticoids. In fact, chronic administration of pharmacologic dosages of glucocorticoids is the most common cause of adrenal insufficiency. This form of adrenal insufficiency is labeled tertiary, in that exogenous glucocorticoids lead to a decrease in corticotropin-releasing hormone (CRH) production and release by the hypothalamus, leading to decreased adrenocorticotropic hormone (ACTH) production by the anterior pituitary, leading to decreased cortisol production by the adrenal gland. Hence, once the exogenous glucocorticoids are withdrawn, especially when sudden, an adrenal crisis of acute cortisol deficiency can ensue, leading to the clinical presentation above.

CASE CONTINUED

The patient was taken to the ICU, where normal saline with glucose was administered IV. Hydrocortisone, 100 mg IV q6h, was empirically administered, given the presumptive diagnosis of adrenal crisis; she was also started empirically on antibiotics, as sepsis could not be definitively ruled out. A.I.'s daughter returned with the Mexican asthma medication package, which was found to be a combination of oral theophylline and prednisone, at a dose equivalent to approximately 10 mg PO QD. The patient's hypotension and electrolyte abnormalities reversed quickly with the above therapy and antibiotics were discontinued after the blood cultures were confirmed negative for 48 hours. The patient was ultimately discharged on a very prolonged steroid taper and osteoporosis workup under the direction of an endocrinologist.

QUESTIONS

121. Primary adrenal failure can be distinguished from secondary adrenal insufficiency most readily by what test?
    A. Cortisol levels
    B. ACTH levels
    C. CRH levels
    D. Presence of hyperkalemia
    E. Dexamethasone suppression test

122. In the syndrome of tertiary adrenal insufficiency described above, what would be the response of the adrenal glands to prolonged exogenous ACTH stimulation?
    A. Progressive increase in cortisol secretion
    B. No or little change in cortisol secretion
    C. Decrease in ACTH production
    D. Increase in ACTH production
    E. Decrease in CRH production

123. Which leukocyte subset is proportionally increased in adrenal insufficiency?
    A. Neutrophils
    B. Lymphocytes
    C. Monocytes
    D. Eosinophils
    E. Basophils

124. Which of the following is *not* a cause of primary adrenal insufficiency?
    A. Autoimmune (idiopathic)
    B. Tuberculosis
    C. Adrenal hemorrhage
    D. HIV infection
    E. Hypoglycemia

CASE 32 / KEEPING THAT SUGAR DOWN

CC/ID: 66-year-old woman with h/o type II DM transferring her care to a new medical provider.

HPI: 66-year-old woman with 10 year h/o type II DM on oral hypoglycemics. H.S. has been unhappy with her previous site of care, feeling that "they were not addressing all the things I know I need as a diabetic" and is transferring her care to your diabetes clinic. Diagnosed with DM 10 years ago after presenting with polyuria and polydipsia and has been fairly well-maintained on oral hypoglycemics since. Her last HBA1C was 9.8; she last saw a podiatrist 2 years ago for foot care. Her only complaints in office today are mild numbness and tingling in her feet bilaterally, and occasional blurriness of vision. She denies fever, chills, night sweats, weight loss, polyuria, polydipsia, rashes, chest pain or SOB. H.S. does not exercise regularly, and eats meat approximately five times a week.

PMHx: Hyperlipidemia. Depression/anxiety disorder.

Meds: Glyburide, 5 mg QD; simvastatin, 10 mg QD; metformin, 500 mg BID; ECASA, 325 mg QD

All: NKDA

SHx: No smoking; drinks a glass of wine once or twice a week; no illicit drugs. Homemaker.

FHx: Mother had type II DM and died of MI age 62; Father has hypertension.

VS: Temp 36.8°C, HR 85, BP 138/87, RR 12, O_2 sat 95% RA

PE: *Gen:* well-appearing, moderately obese woman, no acute distress. *HEENT:* fundal exam reveals proliferation of blood vessels suggestive of diabetic retinopathy; mild corneal opacification bilaterally; vision 20/40 on right, 20/35 on left; TMs clear. *Neck:* no LAN; no JVD; no thyromegaly or masses. *CV:* RRR S_1S_2; no murmurs, gallops, or rubs. *Lungs:* CTA bilaterally. *Abdomen:* soft; +BS; NT/ND; no HSM. *Ext:* bilateral feet without rashes or lesions; mild reduction to sensation to pinprick bilaterally.

Labs: Na 142; K 4.0; Cl 112; HCO_3 28; BUN 25; Cr 1.0; fasting Glu 205; LFTs and CBC WNL; TSH 3.4; UA with 1+ glu; 2+protein; no ketones; HBA1C 9.5; Fasting profiles: Total cholesterol 215; LDL 123; HDL 40; Triglycerides 256.

THOUGHT QUESTIONS
- What are the reasons for strict glycemic control in diabetes mellitus?
- What are the goals of glycemic therapy in type I and II diabetes mellitus?

The largest study of patients with type II diabetes, the United Kingdom Prospective Diabetes Study (UKPDS), demonstrated that improved blood glucose control in patients treated intensively for diabetes reduced the risk of developing retinopathy and nephropathy, and possibly neuropathy. In addition, this study showed a 16% reduction in the risk of combined fatal or nonfatal MI and sudden death in the intensively treated (improved glycemic control) group. The Diabetes Control and Complications Trial (DCCT) conclusively demonstrated that, in patients with type I DM, the risk of development or progression of retinopathy, nephropathy, and neuropathy is reduced 50% to 75% by intensive treatment regimens when compared with conventional treatment regimens. The reduction in risk of these complications correlated continuously with the reduction in HBA1C produced by intensive treatment. The goals of glycemic therapy in patients with diabetes to minimize microvascular complications, based on the studies above, is shown in Table 32.

TABLE 32. Glucose Measurements and HBA1C Values in Diabetics

	NORMAL	GOOD	ADDITIONAL ACTION SUGGESTED
Plasma values (mg/dL)			
Average preprandial glucose	<110	90–130	<90/>150
Average bedtime glucose	<120	110–150	<110/>180
HBA1C	<6	<7	>8

CASE CONTINUED

Given H.S.'s elevated fasting glucose and HBA1C, along with evidence of mild proliferative retinopathy, stricter glycemic control was discussed. Patient was referred to a nutritionist and instructed to check her blood sugars initially four times a day and keep a glucose diary. Her glyburide was increased initially to 10 mg PO QD, metformin to 850 mg PO TID, simvastatin to 20 mg and then 40 mg PO QD for better hyperlipidemic control. Urine was checked for microalbuminuria, which showed a cumulative level of 250 mg/24 hours. An ACE inhibitor was initiated. H.S. was referred to both an ophthalmologist for her retinopathy and a podiatrist for routine foot care and formal neuropathy testing. She was instructed on implementation of a regular exercise program and a weight loss program.

QUESTIONS

125. Which of the following is the most serious side effect of metformin?
    A. Abdominal discomfort
    B. Diarrhea
    C. Lactic acidosis
    D. Hypoglycemia
    E. Weight gain

126. What is the goal for LDL reduction in adult diabetics?
    A. LDL <180 mg/dL
    B. LDL <160 mg/dL
    C. LDL <130 mg/dL
    D. LDL <100 mg/dL
    E. LDL <90 mg/dL

127. What is the goal of hypertension lowering in diabetics?
    A. BP <160/100
    B. BP <150/90
    C. BP <140/90
    D. BP <130/80
    E. BP <120/80

128. Which of the following is *not* considered a major risk factor for type II diabetes?
    A. Obesity
    B. LDL >150 mg/dL
    C. Family history of diabetes
    D. Polycystic ovary syndrome
    E. History of gestational diabetes mellitus or delivery of a baby weighing >9 lbs

CC/ID: 42-year-old woman presents with fever, agitation, and SOB.

HPI: H.T., a 42-year-old woman from the West Indies, with known h/o Graves disease and ongoing IV heroin abuse, was brought to the ER by ambulance after being found on the street, agitated and disheveled. History gleaned from medical records revealed that H.T. has an approximately 3-year history of Graves disease but has been largely noncompliant with antithyroid drugs and has refused radioactive ablation in the past. H.T. has a history of being admitted with symptoms of heroin overdose or hyperthyroidism, but leaving against medical advice once the immediate symptoms resolve. Although she is unable to give a clear history secondary to marked agitation, H.T. admits to not currently taking propylthiouracil as prescribed. She reports fevers and chills for the past 4 days accompanied by severe SOB with minimal exertion. She also reports vomiting and has had severe diarrhea "for a long time." You are unable to ascertain symptoms of heat intolerance, palpitations, weakness, visual changes, skin or hair changes secondary to mental state.

PMHx: Graves disease diagnosed 3 years ago. Drainage of multiple skin abscesses (secondary to IV drug use).

Meds: None per patient. Last hospitalization summary 6 months ago showed that patient had been prescribed propylthiouracil, 200 mg PO QD, and propranolol, 20 mg PO QID prior to leaving AMA.

All: NKDA (per chart)

SHx: Patient unable to answer questions regarding habits but is often brought to ED secondary to heroin overdose or with complications of IV heroin use per chart. No h/o smoking or EtOH. Homeless.

VS: Temp 38.5°C; BP 100/40; HR 140 and irregular; RR 20, O_2 sat 90% on RA; weight 45 kg (lost 10 kg since last admission 6 months ago per hospital records)

PE: *Gen:* agitated, cachectic, chronically ill-appearing black woman with mild respiratory distress, unable to sit still with visible tremor. *HEENT:* lid lag and exophthalmos present; dry mucus membranes. *Neck:* JVD of ~10 cm with HJR; no LAN; diffuse goiter with a bruit heard over thyroid. *CV:* irregularly irregular; S_1S_2; tachy with no murmurs, gallops, or rubs appreciated. *Lungs:* rales bilaterally approximately 1/3 of the way up. *Abdomen:* soft; +BS; diffuse tenderness to palpation without rebound; +voluntary guarding; ND; no HSM. *Ext:* pretibial myxedema bilaterally. *Skin:* warm, flushed, smooth; alopecia present; multiple scars from old abscesses. *Neuro:* Pt unable to cooperate with mental status, strength or sensation testing although clearly agitated and not clearly oriented to time or place; hyperreflexia observed throughout.

Labs: WBC 14.00 with neutrophilic predominance; Hct 31 with MCV 85; Plt 150,000; Na 148; K 3.0; BUN 30; Cr 0.9; glu 220; Ca 10.5; Total bili 1.1; AST 90; ALT 108; Alk phos 180; Alb 3.0; TSH undetectable; Free T_4 72 µg/dL: Urine negative for heroin. *ECG:* Rhythm strip shown below (Figure 33); full ECG also shows nonspecific ST-T changes in anterior leads. *CXR:* diffuse pulmonary edema; no infiltrates.

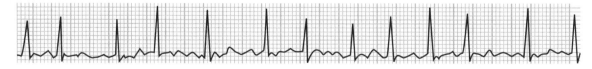

FIGURE 33 Rhythm strip for 42-year-old woman with fever, agitation and SOB. (Illustration by Shawn Girsberger Graphic Design.)

THOUGHT QUESTIONS

- What arrhythmia is present in Figure 33?
- What is the most likely cause of this patient's condition?
- What is the differential diagnosis of her syndrome?

The ECG strip shows atrial fibrillation (here with a rapid ventricular response of ~150). This patient most likely has acute thyroid storm, precipitated by noncompliance with antithyroid medications in the setting of Graves disease. Her symptoms of fever, weight loss, agitation, disorientation, tremulousness, diarrhea, and abdominal pain are all consistent with thyrotoxicosis, as are the signs of atrial fibrillation with resultant heart failure, pretibial myxedema, lid lag and exophthalmos, wide pulse pressure, along with the laboratory findings. In a similar setting with fewer classic features of thyroid storm, the differential diagnosis includes sepsis and intoxication with anticholinergic and adrenergic agents, notably cocaine and amphetamines. Hypoglycemia as well as several withdrawal syndromes (ethanol, narcotics, sedative-hypnotics), may produce a picture of adrenergic hyperfunction and altered mental status, which could be mistaken for hyperthyroidism. Heat stroke, with its characteristic hyperpyrexia and disturbed sensorium, might appear similar to thyrotoxicosis but is usually distinguished by its clinical setting. Patients with psychiatric illness may show signs similar to thyroid hyperactivity.

CASE CONTINUED

H.T. was taken to the ICU and started on propylthiouracil (PTU), potassium iodide, hydrocortisone, propranolol, and broad-spectrum antibiotics. Blood and urine cultures were obtained, which were negative after 48 hours, therefore the antibiotics were discontinued. With the above management, her immediate symptoms resolved and she was maintained on PTU with referral to surgery for thyroidectomy, given her Graves disease in the setting of poor medical compliance. However, H.T. left against medical advice prior to surgical evaluation.

QUESTIONS

129. What is the purpose of the steroids in the management of thyroid storm?
    A. To block the synthesis of thyroid hormone
    B. To block the peripheral conversion of T_4 to T_3
    C. To block the release of thyroid hormone
    D. To suppress inflammation of the thyroid gland

130. Which of the following is one of the most serious side effects of methimazole?
    A. Arthralgias
    B. Gastrointestinal disturbances
    C. Pulmonary fibrosis
    D. Granulocytopenia
    E. Hypothyroidism

131. Which of the following is *true* of the use of antithyroid drugs or radioactive iodine to control thyrotoxicosis in the setting of pregnancy?
    A. Both methimazole and propylthiouracil (PTU) are contraindicated.
    B. Both antithyroid drugs cross the placenta and are of uncertain safety but methimazole is preferred over PTU.
    C. Both cross the placenta and are of uncertain safety but PTU is preferred over methimazole.
    D. Both methimazole and PTU are safe in pregnancy.
    E. Radioactive iodine therapy is the modality of choice in the setting of pregnancy.

132. Which of the following is *not* a typical symptom of apathetic hyperthyroidism?
    A. Heart failure
    B. Cold intolerance
    C. Atrial fibrillation
    D. Weight loss
    E. Depressed mental functioning

CASE 34 / 65-YEAR-OLD WOMAN WHO HASN'T SEEN A DOCTOR RECENTLY

CC/ID: 65-year-old woman who presents for her first exam in 10 years.

HPI: P.M. is a 65-year-old Russian widow, who has come to live with her son and daughter-in-law in the U.S. Her son, a patient of yours, would like you to evaluate his mother, who has not seen a doctor in 10 years. In particular, he is anxious to make sure that she receives good preventative care. She feels well, and denies constitutional symptoms or SOB. The remainder of her ROS is also negative.

PMHx: Hysterectomy 12 years ago. $G_3P_2Tab_1$ **Meds:** None   **All:** NKDA

SHx: Widowed, former subway conductor, with 2 healthy children aged 29 and 30. No significant alcohol, tobacco, or illicit substance use.

FHx: Father died at 59 of MI; had first MI at age 49. Mother died at 78 "in her sleep." Sister with breast cancer.

VS: Temp 37°C, BP 155/95, HR 78, RR 12, Sat O_2 98% RA; weight 140 lbs

PE: *Gen:* well-groomed woman in no distress, speaking through her son. *HEENT:* conjunctivae, sclerae, and funduscopy normal; OP normal. *Neck:* no thyromegaly or adenopathy; JVP flat; 2+ carotid upstrokes no bruits. *Lungs:* clear. *CV:* RRR normal S_1S_2; 2/6 HSM at LLSB. *Abdomen:* soft, NT/ND, no HSM. *Ext:* no arthropathy or rashes. *Neuro:* normal gait, cranial nerves II–XII.

THOUGHT QUESTIONS

- Does anything in this patient's history and examination suggest an underlying health condition?
- What screening tests are indicated in this patient?
- What screening tests are indicated in a man of similar age?

The patient's family history of breast cancer in a first-degree relative and Ob/Gyn history of having had her first term pregnancy at age >35 increase her risk of developing breast cancer. In addition, her father's history of early MI increases her risk of CAD.

The United States Preventive Services Task Force (USPSTF) regularly issues recommendations for immunizations, screening exams and tests, as do other professional organizations, such as the American College of Physicians (ACP) and American Cancer Society (ACS). For *all adults*, the USPSTF recommends blood pressure measurements every 2 years, tetanus/diphtheria booster every 15 to 30 years, and general health counseling at all routine visits. *All adults >50 years of age* should receive annual stool testing for fecal occult blood (FOBT) as well as sigmoidoscopy at regular intervals; in addition to FOBT, the ACS recommends flexible sigmoidoscopy every 5 years, colonoscopy every 10 years, or air contrast barium enema every 5 to 10 years. *All adults >65 years of age* should receive an annual influenza vaccination, and one-time pneumococcal vaccination (to be repeated after 6 years for immunocompromised hosts). *All women* should undergo annual clinical breast examination starting at age 50; annual-semiannual mammography from age 50 to 65; Pap smears every 3 years from the onset of sexual activity (or age 18) through age 65; and serum cholesterol testing every 5 years from age 50 to 65. The ACS recommends a monthly breast self-examination for all women from 20 years of age; breast examination by a provider every 3 years from age 20 to 40 and annually thereafter; and annual mammography starting at age 40. *All men* should receive serum cholesterol testing every 5 years from ages 35 to 65. The ACS adds a digital rectal examination plus prostate serum antigen (PSA) testing at the time of each non-FOBT screening test for colon cancer in men 50 years of age and older. In addition, many clinicians send a one-time panel consisting of electrolytes/BUN/creatinine/glucose, as well as a CBC, and a urinalysis in any patient new to the clinic.

CASE CONTINUED

You administer the patient's immunizations, perform a breast examination, and order a mammogram, fasting lipid profile, CBC, BUN, and creatinine. Her urine dipstick is normal. Before she leaves, you give her three FOBT cards and explain their use.

QUESTIONS

133. The fasting lipid profile shows elevated total cholesterol, with an LDL of 170 (elevated), an HDL below 30 (decreased), and normal triglycerides. You prescribe aspirin and:
    A. A modified diet and increased exercise
    B. An HMG-CoA reductase inhibitor
    C. Gemfibrozil
    D. (B) and (C)
    E. Nothing else

134. In addressing the patient's blood pressure of 155/95, you decide to:
    A. Start clonidine.
    B. Start hydrochlorothiazide (HCTZ).
    C. Start metoprolol.
    D. Recheck the blood pressure in 1 week.

135. One of the three FOBT cards is positive for occult blood. The next step is to:
    A. Refer the patient for sigmoidoscopy.
    B. Repeat the test.
    C. Refer the patient for colonoscopy.
    D. Order an abdominal CT with contrast.

136. Which of the following statements regarding breast cancer prevention is/are true?
    A. Family history of breast cancer in a mother, daughter, or sister is associated with increased risk of breast cancer in the patient, as is the presence of the *BRCA1* or *BRCA2* mutations.
    B. 75% of women with breast cancer have no first-degree female relative with the disease.
    C. A menstrual history is useful when assessing a woman's risk of breast cancer.
    D. Women younger than 50 or older than 65 who are at an increased risk of developing breast cancer may benefit from screening with clinical breast examination and mammography, but there is no evidence to support this.
    E. All of the above.

CASE 35 / CALCULATING CHOLESTEROL

CC/ID: 46-year-old man with hypertension presents for routine screening.

HPI: H.L. presents to primary care physician for a routine follow-up visit. He is generally in good health except for a 5-year history of hypertension. His only complaint is occasional low back pain after vigorous weight training. He has no fevers, chills, cough, SOB, abdominal pain, nausea, vomiting, bowel symptoms, or urinary symptoms. He reports no weight loss or night sweats. He always wears seatbelts; weight-trains once or twice a week, but doesn't regularly obtain cardiovascular exercise; and eats red meat about 4 to 5 times a week.

PMHx: Appendectomy and vasectomy   **Meds:** HCTZ, 25 mg PO QD   **All:** NKDA

SHx: Smokes 1 ppd for past 20 years; 5 to 6 drinks of beer each weekend. Accountant; married with 3 children.

FHx: Father died of MI at age 68; mother has adult-onset diabetes.

VS: Temp 36.8°C, HR 87, BP 142/89, RR 16, weight 210 lbs

PE: *Gen:* moderately obese, well-appearing man in NAD. *HEENT:* No papilledema; OP clear; no xanthomas. *Neck:* no LAN. *CV:* RRR S$_1$S$_2$; no S$_4$; no murmurs or rubs. *Lungs:* CTA bilaterally. *Abdomen:* soft; obese; +BS; NT/ND; no HSM. *Ext:* no peripheral edema.

Labs: CBC, electrolytes and fasting glucose WNL. Fasting cholesterol profile: Total cholesterol 255; LDL 155; HDL 42; Triglycerides 280.

THOUGHT QUESTIONS

- Which measure of the fasting cholesterol profile (total cholesterol, LDL, HDL, or triglycerides) is the primary target of therapy?
- The goal of LDL cholesterol reduction varies depending on the category of risk for coronary artery disease. What are the three categories of risk that modify LDL cholesterol goals?
- Besides "therapeutic lifestyle changes," which pharmacologic agents assist in lowering LDL cholesterol?
- What is the Friedewald equation for calculating LDL from the other parameters and why is it used?

LDL is the primary target of "cholesterol-lowering" therapy, defined as both lifestyle modification and pharmacologic intervention. Epidemiologic studies, animal experiments, and research on genetic forms of hypercholesterolemia all indicate that elevated LDL cholesterol is a major risk factor for CHD (coronary heart disease). Recent clinical trials show that LDL-lowering therapy reduces the risk of developing CHD. The goal of LDL reduction depends on whether the patient already has CHD or is at high risk of developing CHD (Table 35).

TABLE 35. Different Risk Categories for Coronary Heart Disease (CHD) and the Desired LDL Goal for Each

RISK CATEGORY	LDL GOAL (mg/dL)
I. CHD and CHD risk equivalents (other clinical forms of atherosclerotic disease, such as peripheral arterial disease, abdominal aortic aneurysm, symptomatic carotid artery disease; diabetes; multiple risk factors that confer a 10-year risk for CHD >20%)	<100
II. Two or more risk factors for CHD (that confer a 10-year risk for CHD <20%)	<130
III. Zero to one risk factor for CHD	<160

The risk factors for CHD referred to in Table 35 modify LDL goals and are as follows:

1. Cigarette smoking
2. Hypertension (BP ≥140/90 mmHg or on an antihypertensive medication)
3. Low HDL cholesterol (<40 mg/dL)
4. Family history of premature CHD (CHD in male first-degree relative <55 years; CHD in female first-degree relatives <65 years)
5. Age (men ≥45 years; women ≥55 years)

In terms of treatment for an elevated LDL cholesterol, lifestyle modification—such as reduced intake of saturated fat and cholesterol, increased physical activity, and weight control—can be attempted initially, but pharmacologic therapy should be initiated if the risk for CHD is high or if CHD has already developed. The most common agents for LDL lowering include

1. HMG CoA reductase inhibitors, also called statins (lovastatin, pravastatin, fluvastatin, atorvastatin, cerivastatin)
2. Bile acid sequestrants (cholestyramine, colestipol, colesevelam)
3. Nicotinic acid
4. Fibric acids (gemfibrozil, fenofibrate, clofibrate)

Epidemiologic studies to date have all involved calculation of LDL from the other measured cholesterol parameters. Hence, familiarity with this method of calculation (called the Friedewald equation) is useful. The Friedewald equation is

$$LDL = \text{Total cholesterol} - HDL - (\text{Triglyceride}/5)$$

NOTE: The equation is valid only when triglycerides are ≤400 mg/dL.

CASE CONTINUED

H.L. has two risk factors for CHD (smoking and hypertension) and thus falls in category II of LDL reduction (goal <130 mg/dL). He was thus referred to a nutritionist and instructed to reduce intake of fats and cholesterol, increase fiber in his diet, perform cardiovascular exercise once or twice a week and try to reduce his weight. However, H.L.'s repeat fasting cholesterol profile after 3 months was the following: Total cholesterol 240; HDL 40; Triglycerides 250. This gave him a calculated LDL of 150 mg/dL. He was thus started on pravastatin, 20 mg PO QD; his LDL cholesterol 3 months later was 122 mg/dL.

QUESTIONS

137. Which of the following is *not* a secondary cause of dyslipidemia?
    A. Diabetes
    B. Obesity
    C. Obstructive liver disease
    D. Chronic renal failure
    E. Anabolic steroids

138. Which of the following risk factors in a patient gives an LDL goal of <100 mg/dL?
    A. Age (men ≥45 years; women ≥55 years)
    B. Hypertension (BP ≥140/90 or on an antihypertensive)
    C. High triglycerides ≥400 mg/dL
    D. Low HDL cholesterol ≤35 mg/dL
    E. Diabetes

139. Which of the following is considered an emerging risk factor for coronary heart disease?
    A. Chronic streptococcal infection
    B. Low HDL cholesterol
    C. Hypothyroidism
    D. Apolipoprotrein
    E. Peripheral arterial disease

140. Which of the following drugs decreases LDL levels, but *not* triglyceride levels?
    A. Clofibrate
    B. Cholestyramine
    C. Nicotinic acid
    D. Gemfibrozil
    E. Atorvastatin

CC/ID: 43-year-old HIV-positive male presents to Infectious Diseases clinic with fatigue.

HPI: T.F., a 43-year-old HIV-positive male with CD4 260, viral load undetectable on HAART, presents to the Infectious Diseases clinic complaining of general fatigue. He has a long h/o complicated HIV disease including PCP, multiple pneumonias, and salmonellosis in the past, but has been doing well over the past 3 years on antiretroviral therapy. He recently decided to rejoin the workforce after being on disability for many years and started working at a detox center for HIV-positive IV drug users 3 months ago. T.F. has been keeping long hours at work and feels his fatigue is probably secondary to the workload but wants to be "checked out." He denies any fevers, chills, night sweats, weight loss, dizziness, cough, SOB, abdominal pain, diarrhea, constipation, blood in stool, or urinary symptoms. He feels occasional nausea with HIV medications but no vomiting.

PMHx: Diagnosed with HIV in 1989 and has had multiple opportunistic infections as above, with CD4 nadir 35 in 1993. Has been on same antiretroviral regimen for 3 years and has had undetectable viral loads since; PPD negative 3 months ago prior to starting new job.

Meds: d4T, 40 mg PO BID; indinavir, 800 mg PO BID; ritonavir, 100 mg PO BID; 3TC, 150 mg PO BID; Marinol, 2.5 mg PO QD

All: Septra (rash)

SHx: H/o smoking 20 pack years but quit in 1995; drinks 3 to 4 drinks each weekend; no IVDU but smokes marijuana for help with nausea. Homosexual and currently sexually active with monogamous partner.

VS: Temp 36.2°C, BP 125/82, HR 85, RR 12

PE: *Gen:* thin, well-appearing, white man in NAD. *HEENT:* OP clear; no thrush. *Neck:* no LAN. *CV:* RRR S_1S_2; no murmurs, gallops, or rubs *Lungs:* CTA bilaterally. *Abdomen:* Soft; +BS; NT/ND; no HSM. *Ext:* no edema.

Labs: WBC 5.3; Hct 39.5; Plt 230,000; lytes and LFTs WNL; CD4 286; HIV RNA PCR <50 copies/mL; TSH 2.4; PPD reaction of 6 mm

---

THOUGHT QUESTIONS
- What test should be performed next in this patient?
- What are the criteria for tuberculin (PPD) positivity and the risk factors for developing disease?

This patient has met the cutoff criteria of 5 mm for PPD positivity, in the setting of HIV infection. He must first be ruled out for active tuberculosis with a chest x-ray to decide whether he merits treatment for "latent TB infection" (LTBI, formerly called prophylaxis) versus treatment for active TB.

The decision to treat latent TB (or a positive PPD) in certain groups is based on their risk of progression to active disease, which in turn is modified by the immune status of the host and the time since TB exposure. Persons infected with *Mycobacterium tuberculosis* are at the greatest risk of developing disease shortly after infection has occurred. The risk of developing active TB in HIV-infected persons with LTBI is 30 to 50 times the risk of developing active disease in a healthy host. The risk of developing TB disease is 10% over a lifetime for immunocompetent people infected with TB; the risk of developing active TB is 7% to 10% *each year* for people who are dually infected with both M-TB and HIV.

The cutoff for PPD positivity thus varies by patient based on his or her risk factor(s) for development of active TB disease from latent TB infection. Groups who have the highest risk of proceeding to active disease will have the lowest tuberculin positivity cutoff in order to increase the sensitivity of the test and avoid false negatives. Table 36 shows the criteria for PPD positivity for each risk group. The current guidelines from the ATS/CDC can be found at www.cdc.gov/epo/mmwr/preview/mmwrhtml/rr4906a1.htm

TABLE 36. Criteria for Tuberculin Positivity by Risk Group

REACTION >5 MM	REACTION >10 MM OF INDURATION	REACTION >15 MM
HIV positive	Recent immigrants (within the last 5 years) from high prevalence countries	Persons with no risk factors for TB
Recent contacts of TB case patients	Injection drug users	
Fibrotic changes on chest x-ray consistent with prior TB	Residents and employees of the following high-risk congregate settings: prisons and jails, nursing homes and other long-term facilities for the elderly, hospitals and other health care facilities, residential facilities for patients with AIDS, and homeless shelters	
	Mycobacteriology lab personnel	
Patients with organ transplantation and other immunosuppressed patients (receiving the equivalent of >15 mg/day prednisone for 1 month or more)	Persons with the following clinical conditions that place them at high risk: silicosis, diabetes, chronic renal failure, some hematologic disorders (e.g., leukemia or lymphoma), other specific malignancies (e.g., carcinoma of the head or neck and lung), weight loss of >10% of ideal body weight, gastrectomy, and jejunoileal bypass	

CASE CONTINUED

T.F. had a chest x-ray, PA and lateral, which was completely clear. He was placed on isoniazid (INH) for treatment of latent TB infection.

QUESTIONS

141. How long is the duration of isoniazid therapy for treatment of latent TB infection in adults?
    A. 12 months in HIV positive patients; 12 months in HIV negative patients
    B. 9 months in HIV positive patients; 9 months in HIV negative patients
    C. 12 months in HIV positive patients; 9 months in HIV negative patients
    D. 12 months in HIV positive patients; 6 months in HIV negative patients
    E. 9 months in HIV positive patients; 3 months in HIV negative patients

142. Which of the following regimens is not approved for treatment of latent TB infection in HIV negative adults?
    A. INH for 9 months
    B. INH for 6 months
    C. Rifampin for 4 months
    D. Rifampin and PZA for 2 months
    E. PZA for 6 months

143. What is the most severe toxicity observed with isoniazid?
    A. Uveitis
    B. Arrhythmias
    C. Liver toxicity
    D. Nephrotoxicity
    E. Glucose intolerance

144. Which vitamin should be coadministered with INH in patients predisposed to peripheral neuropathy to help prevent that complication?
    A. Vitamin B_1 (thiamine)
    B. Vitamin B_2 (riboflavin)
    C. Folic acid
    D. Vitamin B_6 (pyridoxine)
    E. Vitamin B_{12} (cyanocobalamin)

CC/ID: 45-year-old man presents with an excruciating headache and a fever.

HPI: B.M. was in his usual state of good health until 1 week before admission, when he developed left ear pain. This progressed to include bifrontal headache, sinus congestion, and fever. After receiving an "antibiotic" from his primary care physician 3 days ago, he noted transient improvement. Early this morning, however, his fever and headache returned, and he started to vomit. When the patient became drowsy and confused, his boyfriend brought him to the ED.

PMHx: Seasonal allergies; migraines, HIV negative per partner. **PSHx:** Right ACL repair 10 years ago.

Meds: Erythromycin; acetaminophen. **All:** NKDA

SHx: Lives with boyfriend; delivers parcels for overnight mail service. No cigarettes; no recreational drugs; occasional social EtOH.

VS: Temp 40.0°C, BP 140/90, HR 110, RR 18

PE: *Gen:* diaphoretic, moaning, moderate distress, uncooperative. *HEENT:* PERRLA, EOMI; no conjunctival petechiae; pus in left ear canal obscuring TM, bulging right TM; uncooperative with direct funduscopy. *Neck:* stiff. *Lungs:* clear bilaterally. *CV:* regular, tachy, no murmurs. *Abdomen:* soft, +BS, no HSM. *Ext:* clammy skin; no rashes, trackmarks, or embolic stigmata. *Neuro:* uncooperative with exam.

Labs: Pending.

THOUGHT QUESTIONS

- What conditions would you include in this patient's differential diagnosis?

- The patient already has a peripheral IV line. What diagnostic and therapeutic measures do you want to take, and in what order?

With a fever, headache, and neck stiffness, this patient has acute bacterial meningitis until proven otherwise. Other possible diagnoses include parameningeal bacterial infection, such as an epidural, neck, pharyngeal, or brain abscess; fungal, mycobacterial, or viral meningitis; subarachnoid hemorrhage; CNS malignancy; cerebral vasculitis; endocarditis with embolization to the CNS; or the neuroleptic malignant syndrome. Suspected bacterial meningitis is a medical emergency and requires immediate workup and presumptive therapy. This involves immediately drawing two sets of peripheral blood cultures, performing a lumbar puncture (LP), and starting empiric antimicrobial therapy while waiting for test results.

Two contraindications to performing an LP include (a) the presence of a cellulitis or abscess over the area where you would like to insert the needle, and (b) the possibility of intracerebral mass effect, which could cause brainstem herniation if an LP were performed. If either of these contraindications applies, you should draw blood cultures and start empiric antimicrobial therapy before performing the LP. If the patient has a cellulitis over the L4-5 region, you can ask the neurosurgical or radiology services to perform an LP safely in another spinal region. If you suspect an intracerebral mass, you should obtain a head CT before performing the LP. Traditionally, a nonfocal neurologic exam (which requires a cooperative, conscious patient) and the absence of papilledema were thought to rule out significant mass effect. Now, however, many physicians start antibiotics and obtain a head CT before performing an LP on any patient, regardless of exam findings. CSF obtained 1 to 2 hours after initiation of antibiotics is still likely to yield microbiologic results.

CASE CONTINUED

Because the patient cannot cooperate with the neurologic exam, you draw two peripheral blood cultures, start antibiotics, and obtain a head CT, which shows pansinusitis, but no mass lesions. You perform an LP, and walk the specimen to the microbiology lab. Forty-five minutes later, the microbiology tech calls you down to the lab. You see WBCs and gram-positive, quellung-positive diplococci on the smear of the CSF. The next day, the CSF and blood cultures return *Streptococcus pneumoniae* that is intermediately resistant to penicillin and fully resistant to erythromycin.

QUESTIONS

145. In addition to CSF for bacterial smear and culture, glucose, protein, and cell counts, what tests should you order?
    A.   CSF smear and culture for acid-fast bacilli (AFB)
    B.   CSF smear and culture for fungus
    C.   CSF and serum cryptococcal antigen
    D.   CSF VDRL
    E.   All of the above

146. Which of the following empiric antibiotic regimens should you choose?
    A.   Ampicillin and gentamicin
    B.   Vancomycin and gentamicin
    C.   Ceftriaxone and vancomycin
    D.   Ciprofloxacin and ceftriaxone

147. While you are obtaining the history from the patient's boyfriend, he tells you that the patient once said that he became short of breath after taking penicillin. Your approach to treatment would be to:
    A.   Give ceftriaxone and vancomycin.
    B.   Give vancomycin, add rifampin, and ask the allergy/immunology service to perform urgent skin testing for penicillin allergy and desensitize the patient if testing is positive.
    C.   Give ceftriaxone, vancomycin, and prednisone.
    D.   Give chloramphenicol and vancomycin.

148. If your patient were a 65-year-old presenting with symptoms of meningitis, without the history of otitis media and sinusitis, which of the following antibiotics would you add to your empiric regimen?
    A.   Chloramphenicol
    B.   Ampicillin
    C.   Acyclovir
    D.   Dexamethasone

CASE 38 / STUFFY NOSE

CC/ID: 21-year-old man with h/o allergic rhinitis presents with headache and yellow nasal discharge.

HPI: S.S. is a 21-year-old man generally in good health except for a h/o seasonal allergies. He presents to his family practitioner with a 10 day h/o subjective fevers, severe pain over both cheeks and radiating to his teeth, and purulent nasal discharge. He developed clear nasal congestion along with a sore throat, fatigue, itchy eyes, and sneezing approximately 3 weeks prior to presentation, which he attributed to his allergic rhinitis. However, these symptoms did not clear up with his usual nasal steroid and oral antihistamine, and S.S. reports fevers and chills developing 5 days ago, along with a change in the nasal drainage to yellowish to dark green. The pain in his cheeks and teeth started approximately 4 days ago and is described as an intense, throbbing pressure, worse with leaning forward. S.S. tried OTC decongestants in addition to his usual rhinitis regimen, but felt no change in his condition. He has a sporadic cough, exacerbated by lying supine, which occasionally brings up yellowish mucus. He has no diplopia, SOB, abdominal symptoms, urinary symptoms, joint pains, or rashes. He denies ever having these symptoms previously,

PMHx: Allergic rhinitis; eczema as young child.

Meds: Vancenase nasal spray, 2 sprays to each nostril BID, PRN for congestion; Claritin 10 mg PO QD

All: Sulfa drugs (rash)

SHx: No smoking; no EtOH; no drugs. Patient is studying to be elementary school teacher and is interning with kindergartners.

FHx: Family history of atopy, otherwise noncontributory.

VS: Temp 38.0°C, BP 125/82, HR 70, RR 16, O_2 sat 96% on RA

PE: *Gen:* well-developed, well-appearing man in some pain but NAD. *HEENT:* no edema of the eyelids; severe pain to palpation over the maxillary sinuses and teeth; few nasal polyps; purulent discharge observed draining from turbinates; transillumination reveals impaired light transmission in the maxillary sinuses. Ear examination with bulging, mildly erythematous TM on right side albeit light reflex present; left TM clear. *Neck:* mild shotty anterior cervical LAN. *CV:* RRR S_1S_2; no murmurs, gallops, or rubs. *Lungs:* CTA bilaterally. *Abdomen:* soft; +BS; NT/ND; no HSM. *Ext:* no edema; no clubbing; no rashes.

Labs: WBC 13.00 with neutrophilic predominance, otherwise labs unremarkable.

THOUGHT QUESTIONS

- Are there any diagnoses on the differential that must be ruled out prior to assuming a diagnosis of sinusitis and treating?
- What are some of the methods used to make the diagnosis of bacterial sinusitis?

The symptoms this patient is describing are suggestive of bacterial sinusitis, probably as a result of superinfection after his viral URI. Although viral URIs and allergic or vasomotor rhinitis are the most common causes of sinus symptoms, this syndrome is suggestive of a bacterial process given the fevers, severity of the pain, and purulent nasal discharge. Several conditions produce symptoms resembling sinusitis, including polyps, tumors, cysts, foreign bodies, and vasculitides such as Wegener granulomatosis. The diagnosis of sinusitis is usually a clinical one. The gold standard of sinusitis diagnosis is a positive culture on sinus aspiration, but the invasive nature of the procedure and its low sensitivity and specificity restricts its use to refractory cases. Sinus plain films can show mucosal thickening, sinus opacification, or air-fluid levels, but the sensitivity and specificity are poor. For the maxillary sinusitis, a single occipitomental (Waters) view is acceptable to examine the sinuses, but ethmoid sinuses are best visualized by CT scan. CT is best reserved for complicated disease, search for occult ethmoidal disease, and delineation of anatomy prior to endoscopic surgery.

MRI has proven useful for differentiating mucosal inflammation from tumor. Ultrasound has also been used in the diagnosis of sinusitis, with a higher specificity than sinus x-rays, but a lower sensitivity. Diagnostic nasal endoscopy has been advanced as a primary evaluation strategy in patients with recurrent or chronic symptoms. Endoscopy can be performed in the office by an oto-laryngologist, allowing the physician to perform a more complete examination of the nasopharynx, and to obtain material for bacteriologic examination. None of these studies need be performed in our patient with a routine sinus infection.

QUESTIONS

149. Which one of the following is *not* a risk factor for the development of sinusitis?
    A. Nasal polyps
    B. Deviated nasal septum
    C. Dental abscess
    D. Rapid changes in altitude
    E. Eczema

150. Which of the following is *not* recommended as ancillary treatment for sinusitis?
    A. Antihistamines
    B. Decongestants
    C. Nasal sprays, such as phenylephrine hydrochloride
    D. Expectorants, such as guaifenesin

151. Which of the following antibiotics (if indicated) is recommended as first-line therapy?
    A. Trimethoprim-sulfamethoxazole
    B. Amoxicillin-clavulanate
    C. Amoxicillin
    D. Macrolide
    E. Fluoroquinolone

152. Sinusitis is the primary source of infection in approximately what percentage of patients with intracranial abscesses?
    A. 25%
    B. 33%
    C. 50%
    D. 67%
    E. 75%

CC/ID: 20-year-old man with fever and sore throat for 4 days.

HPI: B.P., a line cook, was well until 4 days ago when he experienced the abrupt onset of burning discomfort in the back of his throat, cervical adenopathy, "mucous" in his mouth, the sensation of fever, and malaise. He took an OTC liquid cold preparation with no relief, but felt transient, partial relief with acetaminophen. He came to your urgent care clinic because he was experiencing discomfort when swallowing, and because he wasn't getting any better. He is able to swallow and denies difficulty handling his oral secretions. He also complains of mild headache and myalgias. He denies sinus congestion, cough, SOB, nausea, vomiting, and diarrhea. He denies sex without condoms, intravenous drug use, and transfusions. He can't remember any recent sick contacts.

PMHx: Fractured right arm as a child, no sequelae. Denies major illnesses, hospitalizations.

Meds: Acetaminophen PRN **All:** No known allergies.

SHx: Emigrated from Mexico 2 years ago. Shares an apartment with friends. No cigarettes; occasional EtOH and marijuana. In monogamous relationship with girlfriend; they use condoms.

VS: Temp 39°C, BP 130/70, HR 100, RR14, Sat O_2 99% RA

PE: *Gen:* well-developed man in some discomfort but no distress, able to speak in a normal voice. *HEENT:* normal funduscopy, nasal turbinates, TMs. Erythematous pharynx, with whitish tonsillar exudates. Uvula midline. No bulging masses. No ulcers or vesicles. *Neck:* supple, tender bilateral cervical adenopathy. *Lungs:* clear bilaterally. *CV:* RRR, normal S_1S_2, flow murmur. *Abdomen:* soft, no upper quadrant tenderness or hepatosplenomegaly. *Skin:* no rashes or nodules. *Ext:* warm, well perfused, no arthropathies.

THOUGHT QUESTIONS

- What organism do you think is causing this patient's pharyngitis?
- Can you tell from the examination?

This 20-year-old man presents with fever and pharyngitis of 4 days' duration. The most likely bacterial pathogen is group A beta-hemolytic *Streptococcus*. Other possible bacteria include *Neisseria gonorrhoeae, Chlamydia* sp, *Corynebacterium diptheriae*, anaerobic streptococci, or *Mycoplasma*. Possible viral pathogens include rhinovirus, coronavirus adenovirus, parainfluenza, coxsackie A or B, HSV 1 or 2, EBV, or HIV. Classic pharyngitis caused by group A *Streptococcus* is said to produce a clinical syndrome of pharyngitis, purulent exudates, fever, cervical lymphadenopathy, and leukocytosis; however, this is nonspecific enough to apply to many of the agents listed above. Definitive diagnosis requires culture. The presence of vesicles would point toward infection with coxsackie A virus or primary HSV. Hepatosplenomegaly would suggest EBV infection (mononucleosis). The presence of myalgias and a maculopapular rash on the chest and back would be concerning for primary HIV infection.

CASE CONTINUED

You readdress the possibility of HIV infection, and the patient repeatedly denies high-risk behavior in the last 6 months. A CBC shows 15,000 WBC, mostly PMNs.

QUESTIONS

153. You strongly doubt EBV, HIV, and HSV infection. Your initial diagnostic and therapeutic strategy should be:
    A. Benzathine penicillin IM × 1; or penicillin V, 500 mg PO BID × 10 days
    B. Rapid streptococcal agglutination test; penicillin if positive, no treatment if negative
    C. Throat culture; culture-directed antibiotics if positive, no treatment if negative
    D. Rapid streptococcal agglutination test; penicillin if positive, culture and directed antibiotic therapy if negative.
    E. (A), (C), or (D).

154. The two most important reasons for treating this patient for group A *Streptococcus* are:
    A. To shorten the duration of symptoms to less than 1 week
    B. To prevent local complications of streptococcal infection
    C. To prevent renal disease, arthritis, and endocarditis
    D. (A) and (B)
    E. (B) and (C)

155. Three days after seeing you, the patient pages you to say that he is not feeling any better. His culture was positive for group A *Streptococcus*, and he has been taking the antibiotics you prescribed. You tell him:
    A. "Give the antibiotics a few more days to work."
    B. "Stop taking penicillin and start taking ciprofloxacin."
    C. "Come to my office this morning so I can take a look."
    D. "Go directly to the emergency department."

156. Imagine a different scenario, in which the patient reports recently performing oral sex. The culture is pending. The patient denies systemic symptoms, and the rest of the physical exam is negative. You decide to treat for gonococcal pharyngitis with:
    A. Penicillin and doxycycline
    B. Penicillin
    C. Doxycycline
    D. Ceftriaxone, 125 mg IM, and doxycycline

CC/ID: 23-year-old woman athlete generally in good health presents with bleeding gums.

HPI: 23-year-old woman presents to Urgent Care clinic complaining of a 4-week history of gum bleeding during teeth brushing. I.T. has generally been in good health except for a prolonged viral URI about 2 months prior to presentation. She did not seek medical attention at the time, but took OTC medication with eventual resolution. Approximately 1 month ago, I.T. noticed that routine brushing of her teeth yielded spontaneous bleeding from her gums. She has had no recent dental procedures, does not floss, and has no known gum disease. Of note, she has never had any bleeding problems before. Patient denies any fever, chills, night sweats, weight loss, cough, SOB, headache, visual changes, abdominal pain, nausea, vomiting, or changes in urinary patterns. She does report a longer menstrual period than usual 2 weeks ago with 5 days of heavy bleeding (usual pattern is 2 days of heavy bleeding), necessitating the use of about 8 pads per day for those 5 days. Also reports bruises and "spider rashes" on her lower legs, which she attributes to trauma from sports activities, and severe "freckling" on shoulders, which she attributes to sun exposure. I.T. denies any epistaxis, hematuria or blood in stool. She has not noticed prolonged bleeding with cuts but has not cut herself in recent memory. She denies any sick contacts, travel, or animal exposure. Only new medication she is taking is one that she borrowed from her soccer coach "to take at night to help my leg cramping go away."

PMHx: H/o tibial-plateau fracture right leg 2 years ago s/p ORIF (no bleeding problems during surgery). H/o pneumonia as child.

Meds: Multivitamins and protein supplements. Took approximately 10 doses of a medication from her coach for leg cramps. Phone call to family member identifies the pill as "quinine sulfate."

All: Codeine (patient reports "major mental disconnect" from taking codeine after surgery)

SHx: No smoking; no EtOH; no drugs or IVDU. Patient is professional athlete, formerly a gymnast and now a soccer player. Patient has never been sexually active, and lives with parents.

FHx: No h/o bleeding disorders or blood malignancies in family.

VS: Temp 36.9°C, BP 105/65, HR 55, RR 12, O_2 sat 99% RA

PE: *Gen:* well-appearing, muscular young woman in NAD. *HEENT:* no conjunctival hemorrhages; scattered petechiae in the posterior OP; spontaneous bleeding from gums with mild probing; no findings of gingivitis. *Neck:* no LAN; no JVD; supple; shoulders with multiple scattered minute, red to purple petechial hemorrhages, nonblanching. *CV:* RRR S_1S_2; no murmurs, gallops, or rubs. *Lungs:* CTA bilaterally. *Abdomen:* Soft; +BS; NT/ND; no hepatomegaly; ?spleen tip palpable. *Rectal:* deferred because of concern about bleeding but stool tested after BM and was found to be brown but guaiac-positive. *Ext:* multiple scattered petechiae over lower extremities with a few scattered ecchymoses.

Labs: WBC 6.0; Hct 41.0; Plt 12.000; LFTs, lytes, coag profiles all WNL.

THOUGHT QUESTIONS
- What is the differential diagnosis of this patient's condition?
- What is the initial diagnostic step for any patient with this condition?

This patient has an isolated thrombocytopenia, with the differential diagnosis easily generated from considering disorders of decreased platelet production and increased platelet destruction (with consideration of artifactual reasons for observation of thrombocytopenia). In terms of disorders of increased platelet destruction, the list can be divided into immunologic processes (autoimmune and alloimmune), nonimmunologic processes (basically divided into the microangiopathic processes and traumatic shearing), and abnormal platelet pooling. In terms of decreased platelet production, thrombopoiesis can be ineffective from a number of acquired and hereditary disorders. The first step in evaluating any hematologic profile disorder is to evaluate the blood smear. Artifactual reasons (e.g., clumping) for thrombocytopenia can be evaluated on the blood smear; decreased platelet production and immunologic destruction of platelets will both result in a dearth of platelets on the blood smear; microangiopathic processes of destruction reveal very specific blood smear findings (e.g., schistocytes, target cells).

CASE CONTINUED

Blood smear showed a paucity of platelets with a few giant platelets observed. No schistocytes; no abnormalities of the red blood cells or white cells.

QUESTIONS

157. Which of the following is I.T.'s most likely diagnosis based on the history and the blood smear?
    A. Thrombotic thrombocytopenic purpura (TTP)
    B. Hereditary thrombocytopenia
    C. Platelet satellitism
    D. Immune-mediated thrombocytopenia (ITP)
    E. Disseminated intravascular coagulation

158. Which of the following would be usually elevated in ITP?
    A. LDH
    B. PT and PTT
    C. Fibrinogen
    D. Antiplatelet antibodies
    E. Creatinine

159. Which of the following drugs is *not* associated with the development of ITP?
    A. Heparin
    B. Sulfonamides
    C. Amiodarone
    D. Quinine/quinidine
    E. Alcohol

160. Which of the following is the initial therapy for ITP?
    A. Splenectomy
    B. Fresh frozen plasma transfusions
    C. Plasmapheresis
    D. Platelet transfusions
    E. Glucocorticoids

CASE 41 / 50-YEAR-OLD MAN WITH FATIGUE AND NOSEBLEED

CC/ID: 50-year-old male complains of fatigue and recurrent nosebleeds for 3 weeks.

HPI: A.L. presents to the ED with recurrent nosebleeds. He was in his usual state of health until approximately 3 weeks ago, when he began to notice unusual fatigue, which he initially ascribed to the summer heat. In the last 5 days, he has also noted mild exertional tachypnea. In the last 2 days, he has had four nosebleeds. Noting that he appeared paler than usual, his wife brought him to the ED for evaluation. He denies fevers, chills, cough, chest pain, nausea, vomiting, diarrhea, and joint pain.

PMHx: Noncontributory.   **Meds:** None   **All:** NKDA.

SHx: Married; 2 adult children. Vegetable farmer for 30 years. Quit smoking 10 years ago; occasional EtOH.

VS: Temp 37.7°C, BP 145/75, HR 110, RR 16, O_2 sat 98% RA

PE: *Gen:* somewhat pale, well-developed man in no distress. *HEENT:* dried blood in nares; normal teeth and gums; oral mucosa pale. *Neck:* supple; no adenopathy; normal carotids and JVP; no thyromegaly. *Lungs/chest:* CTA; mild rib tenderness to deep palpation. *Back:* no vertebral point tenderness. *CV:* RRR, normal S_1S_2, no murmurs. *Abdomen:* soft, NT/ND, no HSM. *Skin:* pale, without purpura or petechiae. *Ext:* no clubbing; nail beds pale; no adenopathy. *Neuro:* AO×3, CN normal.

Labs: WBC 55,000; Hct 24; Plt 25,000; Lytes normal; Cr 1.0; glucose 95. PT 18 sec; aPTT 45 sec; UA unremarkable. *CXR:* no infiltrates, masses, cardiomegaly, or vertebral lesions.

THOUGHT QUESTIONS
- Summarize this patient's presentation.
- What is the differential diagnosis of a WBC count of 55,000?
- What one test would you order to help with the diagnosis?

This 50-year-old man presents with fatigue, pallor, epistaxis of 3 weeks' duration, anemia, thrombocytopenia, an elevated WBC count, and prolonged PT and PTT. The differential diagnosis of an elevated WBC includes infection, leukemoid reaction, mononucleosis, or leukemia. The combination of anemia, thrombocytopenia, and an abnormal WBC count of recent onset is particularly worrisome for acute leukemia, which is caused by the unregulated proliferation of an immature hematopoietic cell. The progeny of this cell, called blasts, crowd out normal RBC, WBC, and platelets from the bone marrow and peripheral blood, leading to the typical presentation of pancytopenia with circulating blasts. Patients with acute leukemia are therefore at high risk of hemorrhagic and infectious complications, as well as certain metabolic abnormalities particular to several disease subtypes.

Definitive diagnosis is made by bone marrow biopsy, which is subjected to morphological, immunohistochemical, and cytogenetic testing to determine the presence of acute lymphocytic leukemia (ALL) versus acute myelogenous leukemia (AML), as well as the subtype, which has implications for prognosis and treatment. However, 90% of patients with acute leukemia will have circulating blasts on peripheral blood smear. If leukemia is suspected on the basis of symptoms and blood counts, the smear should be inspected for the presence of blasts, which would require both urgent hematologic consultation as well as surveillance for hemorrhagic, infectious, and metabolic complications. Acute leukemia is a complicated, rapidly progressive disease that is fatal if untreated, and requires the attention of a hematologic oncologist.

CASE CONTINUED

The patient's smear shows that 40% of the WBCs are, indeed, blasts. You page the hematology/oncology fellow, and start to admit the patient.

QUESTIONS

161. In addition to the laboratory measurements discussed above, all of the following should be determined *except*:
    A. Serum uric acid
    B. Fibrinogen, fibrin split products (FSP), and D-dimer
    C. Absolute neutrophil count (ANC)
    D. Liver transaminases
    E. Iron studies

162. The ANC is 400, the fibrinogen is slightly decreased, the FSP is elevated, and the liver transaminases and uric acid are normal. Overnight, the patient develops a temperature of 38.7°C. As far as the fever is concerned, your approach should be to:
    A. Draw blood and urine cultures and wait for results to begin culture-directed therapy.
    B. Pan culture and start empiric broad-spectrum antibiotic coverage.
    C. Observe, as the fever is consistent with the presentation of leukemia.
    D. (A) or (C).

163. As far as the elevated PT, PTT, and FSP, and decreased fibrinogen levels and platelets are concerned, you should consider:
    A. Transfusion of irradiated platelets
    B. Transfusion of fresh frozen plasma and cryo-precipitate
    C. Heparin
    D. Close observation
    E. All of the above

164. If the patient's blast count were >150,000/μL, you should consider all of the following interventions *except*:
    A. Leukapheresis
    B. Hydroxyurea
    C. Allopurinol and hydration
    D. Plasmapheresis

CC/ID: 51-year-old man with left leg pain.

HPI: A.D. has a long history of IV heroin use and reports that he missed a vein in his left leg while injecting 3 days ago. After local erythema and tenderness developed, he came to the ED for treatment of what he suspected was an abscess. He reports several similar events in the past. On ROS, he also complained of general fatigue during the last year, but denied shaking chills, night sweats, headache, cough, chest pain, nausea, vomiting, diarrhea, or joint pain. He says that his clothes do not fit him any differently than they did 6 months ago.

PMHx: HCV Ab pos; HBV sAb pos, sAg neg; HIV neg 3 months ago.　**Meds:** None　**All:** NKDA

SHx: Daily heroin by injection for "years"; 1 ppd cigarettes for 20 yrs; rare EtOH. Lives with female partner; works as a day-laborer.

VS: Temp 38.3°C, BP 150/85, HR 100, RR 12, O_2 sat 98% RA

PE: *Gen:* thin, chronically ill-appearing man in NAD. *HEENT:* normal direct funduscopy; normal OP, tongue, and lips; poor dentition. *Neck:* supple; no thyromegaly; 2+ carotid upstrokes no bruits. *Lungs:* CTA. *CV:* tachy, regular rhythm; normal S_1S_2 no murmurs or rubs. *Abdomen:* soft, NT/ND; no HSM. *Rectal:* normal tone; smooth, nontender prostate; guaiac-negative. *Ext:* warm, red, tender fluctuance over the medial right calf; trackmarks on both arms. No adenopathy, joint abnormalities, or bone tenderness. *Neuro:* grossly nonfocal.

Labs: Hct 34%; Hgb 11.5 g/dL; MCV 90fL; WBC 12,000; Plt 250,000; Cr 0.8; AST 75; ALT 90; UA unremarkable. *CXR:* no infiltrates, cardiomegaly, or vertebral abnormalities. Diagnostic procedure: needle aspiration of the fluctuant area yields pus.

THOUGHT QUESTIONS

- Are you concerned about the hematocrit?
- If so, how would you further evaluate it?

This 51-year-old man's primary illness consists of a fever and an abscess in the setting of injection drug use. In addition, he complains of long-standing fatigue, and has an abnormally low hematocrit and hemoglobin. A hematocrit <41% in men or <37% in women (or a correspondingly low hemoglobin) indicates anemia. Anemia should be considered whenever a patient presents with fatigue, exertional tachypnea, tachycardia, palpitations, or certain skin and mucosal changes, such as mucosal or nail bed pallor, brittle nails, cheilosis, or a smooth tongue. Often, however, less severe anemia is detected as an abnormal lab value during the workup of another primary illness; to ignore it is to miss the diagnosis of an underlying, potentially treatable condition.

Classifying anemia by mean corpuscular volume (MCV) and pathophysiology (increased destruction versus decreased production) helps to narrow its many possible causes. Causes of microcytic (small MCV) anemia include iron deficiency, anemia of chronic disease (ACD), and the thalassemias. Causes of macrocytic (large MCV) anemia include vitamin B_{12} and folate deficiencies, myelodysplasias and chemotherapy, hypothyroidism, and reticulocytosis. A "normocytic" mean corpuscular volume may mask concurrent microcytic and macrocytic anemias. A low reticulocyte count would suggest decreased RBC production, while the morphology of cells on the peripheral smear and elevated LDH and total bilirubin would suggest increased RBC destruction. Anemias caused by decreased RBC production include those due to impaired hemoglobin synthesis (iron deficiency, thalassemia, ACD); impaired DNA synthesis (vitamin B_{12}, folate deficiencies); and bone marrow failure or infiltration (aplasia, leukemia, metastases, infection). Anemias caused by increased RBC destruction include those due to blood loss, intrinsic hemolysis (sickle-cell disease, G6PD deficiency, spherocytosis), and extrinsic hemolysis (antibody-mediated, TTP/HUS, prosthetic heart valve, clostridial infection, hypersplenism). Using the MCV, reticulocyte count, ferritin level, and peripheral blood smear early in the workup of anemia can narrow the range of possible diagnoses and prevent ordering unnecessary tests.

CASE CONTINUED

While patient is hospitalized for observation, blood cultures, and abscess drainage, you decide to work up his anemia.

QUESTIONS

165. All of the following lab values are consistent with iron-deficiency anemia *except*:
    A. Low ferritin
    B. Low transferrin iron binding capacity (TIBC)
    C. High TIBC
    D. Normal MCV
    E. Low MCV

166. The usual treatment of iron deficiency anemia is:
    A. Iron sulfate, 325 mg PO TID, until 3 to 6 months after normalization of hematological lab values
    B. Blood transfusion
    C. Iron sulfate, 325 mg PO TID, until hemato-logic lab values normalize
    D. Dietary modification

167. All of the following lab values would be consistent with anemia of chronic disease *except*:
    A. Normal to slightly low MCV
    B. Normal reticulocyte count
    C. Normal to high ferritin
    D. High TIBC

168. The patient's reticulocyte count and ferritin are normal, and his smear is unremarkable. The TIBC and serum iron are both low. His anemia is most likely due to:
    A. GI blood loss from an occult colon cancer
    B. Hemolysis from clostridial sepsis acquired by injecting
    C. Chronic HCV infection
    D. Renal failure

CC/ID: 39-year-old man brought to ER by ambulance with fever and confusion.

HPI: 39-year-old man previously in good health with 2 weeks of general weakness and fatigue per wife. A week prior to admission, L.P. began developing low-grade fevers, which he attributed to a cold. Wife also noted L.P. bleeding from gums when brushing his teeth over the past week, along with "bruising" on his lower legs. On the day of admission, L.P.'s wife found him on the bathroom floor, holding his head and muttering. L.P. was not able to answer simple questions, and his wife called an ambulance. He has no facial droop; speech is clear; no apparent weakness of any extremities. His wife says he has no recent reported abdominal pain, nausea, vomiting, diarrhea, or urinary symptoms.

PMHx: None   **Meds:** None   **All:** NKDA

SHx: Works as engineer; married with 4 children <10 years old. No smoking; no EtOH; no drugs.

VS: Temp 38.2°C, BP 128/73, HR 110, RR 16, O$_2$ sat 95% RA

PE: *Gen:* somnolent-appearing man, pale, mildly jaundiced. *Neuro:* somnolent and oriented only to name; couldn't name place or date; could follow simple commands; nonfocal. *HEENT:* icteric sclera; dried blood around lower gums; petechial rash in posterior palate. *Neck:* no LAN. *CV:* RRR S$_1$S$_2$; tachy; no murmurs, gallops, or rubs. *Lungs:* CTA bilaterally. *Abdomen:* soft; +BS; diffuse abdominal pain to palpation; no rebound or guarding; ND; no hepatomegaly; spleen tip palpable. *Ext:* nonpalpable small purpuric lesions and scattered petechiae over lower extremities; no joint abnormalities.

Labs: WBC 9.5 with 79% neutrophils and 14% bands; Hct 28; Plt count 15,000; Total bili 7.0 (direct 0.8) AST 105; ALT 59; Alk phos 125; LDH 985; PT/PTT within normal limits. Fibrinogen and fibrin split products WNL; BUN 55; Cr 1.2; UA positive for 1+ protein; 2+ blood; negative leukocyte esterase. HIV Ab test negative. Blood smear (Figure 43). *Micro:* blood cultures × 2 negative; Urine culture negative. *ECG:* NSR and unremarkable; *CXR:* clear. *Head CT:* negative for intracranial bleed.

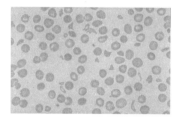

FIGURE 43 Blood smear reveals fragmented red blood cells (schistocytes). Can also typically see nucleated RBCs, basophilic stippling, and sparse platelets in this syndrome. (Copyrighted material is used with permission of Edward C. Klatt, and WebPath, www.medlib.med.utah.ed/WebPath.)

THOUGHT QUESTIONS

- What is the differential diagnosis for the findings on this patient's blood smear?
- What is the most likely diagnosis for this particular patient?

This patient's blood smear reveals schistocytes, or RBC fragments, a finding characteristic of the syndrome of microangiopathic hemolytic anemia (MAHA). MAHA designates any hemolytic anemia related to red cell fragmentation occurring in association with small vessel disease. RBC fragmentation can also be observed in a blood smear secondary to shearing or mechanical fragmentation from disorders of the heart or great vessels. The differential for schistocytes or RBC fragmentation on a blood smear (along with accompanying thrombocytopenia) is shown in Table 43.

TABLE 43. Disorders of Microangiopathic Hemolytic Anemia and Thrombocytopenia
Small vessel disease Thrombotic thrombocytopenic purpura (TTP) Hemolytic uremic syndrome (HUS) Disseminated intravascular coagulation (DIC, e.g., seen in sepsis) Malignant hypertension Disseminated carcinoma (seen most often with breast, stomach, lung, and pancreas) Pregnancy and postpartum period (e.g., HELLP, eclampsia, and preeclampsia syndromes) Some vasculitis syndromes (e.g., SLE, polyarteritis nodosa, scleroderma, Wegener, systemic amyloidosis) Chemotherapy (mitomycin C, cisplatin, bleomycin) March hemoglobinuria Hemangioma syndromes (e.g., giant hemangioma or Kasabach-Merritt syndrome, cavernous hemangioma)
Mechanical shearing Mechanical or bioprosthetic valves Unoperated valvular disease Coarctation of the aorta

Thrombotic thrombocytopenic purpura (TTP) is a syndrome characterized by disseminated thrombotic occlusions of the microcirculation and is usually described by the pentad of microangiopathic hemolytic anemia, thrombocytopenia, fever, neurologic symptoms, and renal dysfunction. L.P. has the initial four findings of TTP, the most likely diagnosis. Hemolytic uremic syndrome (HUS) is closely related to TTP, but renal findings predominate, neurologic findings are rare, and this syndrome usually occurs in children. L.P. has no mechanical reasons for erythrocyte shearing, is not clinically septic, and has no signs or symptoms of disseminated cancer or vasculitides.

CASE CONTINUED

L.P.'s condition was diagnosed as TTP on clinical grounds, and he was started on plasmapheresis at a tertiary care center within 3 hours of presentation to the ER. Patient continued to receive exchange plasmapheresis every day, but he became progressively obtunded. Multiple salvage therapies were attempted, including splenectomy, but the patient died on the tenth day following admission to the ER. Autopsy revealed massively disseminated thrombotic occlusions of the terminal arterioles and capillaries.

QUESTIONS

169. Which lab test is almost universally elevated in the syndrome of TTP?
    A. Platelets
    B. PTT
    C. Fibrin split products
    D. LDH
    E. GGT

170. Prior infection with which organism is commonly associated with the syndrome of HUS?
    A. *Haemophilus influenzae*
    B. *Escherichia coli* 0157:H7
    C. *Campylobacter*
    D. Gram-negative organisms
    E. *Staphylococcus aureus*

171. Treatment for TTP includes all but the following:
    A. Plasmapheresis
    B. Intravenous immunoglobulin
    C. Steroids
    D. Splenectomy
    E. Infusions of fresh frozen plasma

172. The incidence of TTP is rising, presumably because of its association with which disease?
    A. HIV disease
    B. Sepsis
    C. Aortic stenosis
    D. Pregnancy
    E. Glioblastoma

CC/ID: 24-year-old man presents to the ER with high fever, rash, and sore throat.

HPI: H.V. is generally in good health, but presents to the ER with a 4-day history of fever, diffuse rash over trunk and extremities, and sore throat. On the day following the onset of fever 4 days ago, he noticed a diffuse erythematous rash over his trunk, arms, and legs, described as nonpruritic and nonpainful. H.V. also describes a severely sore throat, with pain exacerbated by talking or swallowing, as well as diffuse myalgias and arthralgias and profound weakness. He denies any night sweats, coryza, ear pain, neck stiffness, headache, cough, SOB, abdominal pain, nausea, vomiting, diarrhea or constipation, urinary symptoms, or joint pains. He denies any sick contacts, recent travel, recent camping or activities in woods, new medications, or new drugs. He has a cat at home but no other animal exposures.

PMHx: H/o anal warts, h/o syphilis treated 4 years ago, h/o tonsillectomy 6 years ago.

Meds: None   **All:** NKDA

SHx: Smokes "socially" approximately 6 cigarettes each week; drinks about 3 to 4 drinks of hard liquor every Friday and Saturday; smokes marijuana regularly but no IV drug abuse. Has sex with men only and has recently entered a relationship with new boyfriend. Tries to use condoms regularly but not always consistent. Works in a start-up computer company.

VS: Temp 39.0°C, BP 120/69, HR 110, RR 12, O_2 sat 96% on RA

PE: *Gen:* ill-appearing young man, *HEENT:* conjunctiva mildly injected; TMs clear bilaterally; moderate erythema of posterior pharynx without exudates; small 0.5×1 cm clean-based ulceration on right buccal mucosa. *Neck:* supple; moderate lymphadenopathy anterior cervical chain bilaterally and shotty axillary LAN bilaterally. *CV:* RRR S_1S_2; tachy; no murmurs, gallops, or rubs. *Lungs:* CTA bilaterally. *Abdomen:* soft; +BS; NT/ND; no HSM. *Ext:* no edema, no joint abnormalities. *Skin:* diffuse erythematous maculopapular rash scattered over trunk, back, upper and lower extremities, sparing face, palms, and soles. *GU:* normal external genitalia; no urethral discharge; no genital lesions; mild inguinal lymphadenopathy bilaterally.

Labs: WBC 3.50 with normal differential; Hct 44.0; Plt 100,000. Lytes within normal limits; total bili 1.1; AST 78; ALT 90; Alk phos 120; Albumin 4.2.

THOUGHT QUESTIONS

- What is this patient's differential diagnosis?
- What are some additional tests that can be performed to narrow the diagnosis?

The patient's differential diagnosis is vast as he presents with a number of nonspecific signs and symptoms, including fever, rash, pharyngitis, lymphadenopathy, oral ulceration, myalgias, arthralgias, with laboratory analysis revealing leukopenia and mildly elevated liver enzymes. The most likely causes of a systemic process with these symptoms are either infectious, autoimmune, or a drug reaction. Possible infectious causes include viral syndromes, including primary Epstein-Barr or CMV infection, primary HSV infection, acute hepatitis A or B infection, human herpes virus-6 (roseola), acute HIV infection or rubella; bacterial infections such as secondary syphilis, severe (streptococcal) pharyngitis, leptospirosis, meningococcemia, disseminated gonococcal infection or brucellosis; and protozoal diseases such as acute toxoplasmosis or malaria. Less likely is an acute presentation of a rheumatologic illness, such as systemic lupus erythematosus.

Further tests to exclude infectious causes should include blood cultures, monospot and EBV titers, acute CMV titers, hepatitis A IgM and IgG, hepatitis B surface antigen, HBeAg, HBcAb and HB surface antibody, HIV antibody and HIV viral load, RPR and FTA-ABS for syphilis, and Toxo IgM and IgG. An initial nonspecific screening ANA can be performed for possible autoimmune processes.

CASE CONTINUED

Multiple tests were performed: Blood cultures × 3 negative; monospot and acute EBV titers negative; HepA IgM negative, HepA IgG positive; HepBsAg, HepBeAg both negative, HepBsAb and HepBcoreAb both positive, HIV antibody negative, HIV RNA by PCR >100,000 copies/mL; RPR negative, FTA-ABS positive; Toxo IgM negative, Toxo IgG positive; ANA 1:40 with speckled pattern.

QUESTIONS

173. This constellation of symptoms is most likely explained by:
    A. Acute hepatitis B infection
    B. Infectious mononucleosis
    C. Acute presentation of SLE
    D. Acute HIV syndrome
    E. Secondary syphilis

174. Which of the following tests would be positive in acute HIV syndrome?
    A. Anti-EBV nuclear antigen test (EBNA)
    B. VDRL
    C. p24 antigen
    D. Anti-double stranded DNA Ab
    E. Cryoglobulins

175. What is the appropriate *initial* clinical management for this patient's syndrome?
    A. Referral to specialty clinic with possibility of starting appropriate antiviral therapy
    B. Symptomatic therapy only
    C. Hepatitis B IgG and hepatitis B vaccination
    D. NSAIDs and prednisone
    E. Benzathine penicillin 1.2 million units IM × 1

176. In the setting of acute EBV syndrome, administration of which antibiotic is associated with an almost 100% incidence of rash?
    A. Tetracycline
    B. Trimethoprim-sulfamethoxazole
    C. Erythromycin
    D. Amoxicillin
    E. Ciprofloxacin

CC/ID: 31-year-old woman presents to the ER with 4-day h/o nausea and vomiting.

HPI: 31-year-old woman previously in good health presents to the ER with a 4-day h/o severe nausea and vomiting. R.F. has been unable to keep down even liquids secondary to profound nausea. She also reports general fatigue and weakness over the past week and a 2-day h/o swelling in her lower legs, face, and arms. She denies any fevers or chills, but does report feeling feverish approximately 2 weeks ago in the setting of a severe sore throat, with both symptoms resolving after a few days. She has no cough but does describe mild SOB with exertion over the past week. No abdominal pain, diarrhea, or constipation. R.F. has no dysuria but does note that urine has been small in volume and brownish in color. She reports no new medications; no changes in diet; no one sick at home; she does work in an elementary school and "catches everything the kids and their dogs have."

PMHx: Depression.   **All:** NKDA

Meds: Celexa, 20 mg PO QD; oral contraceptive pills

SHx: No smoking; minimal EtOH intake; no IVDU or drugs. Kindergarten teacher; sexually active with monogamous male partner; HIV test negative 2 months prior to admission.

VS: Temp 36.2°C, BP 155/95, HR 85, RR 16, O_2 sat 94% RA

PE: *Gen:* ill-appearing young woman with swollen facies. *HEENT:* mild facial edema; OP clear; no pharyngeal edema or erythema. *Neck:* no LAN; JVD to 9 cm. *CV:* RRR S_1S_2; no murmurs, gallops, or rubs. *Lungs:* crackles bilateral lower lung fields. *Abdomen:* soft; +BS; mildly and diffusely tender to palpation; ND; no HSM. *Ext:* 2+ pitting edema bilateral LE and 1+edema in hands; no rashes; no joint abnormalities.

Labs: WBC 6.4; Hct 35.0; Plt 280,000; Na 130; K 5.9; Cl 110; HCO_3 18; BUN 104; Cr 5.4; Ca 7.0; Phos 4.2; Mg 2.0; LFTs WNL; UA with 3+ protein, granular casts, RBCs, RBC casts and WBCs. *UA:* Figure 45. *Micro:* blood cultures × 2 negative; urine culture negative. *ECG:* NSR; T waves slightly peaked but no PR or QRS widening. *CXR:* mild pulmonary edema.

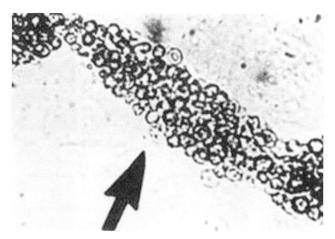

FIGURE 45 Example of RBC cast found in urine sediment. (Copyrighted material is used with permission of the author, the University of Iowa and Virtual Hospital, www.vh.org.)

THOUGHT QUESTIONS
- What process does the urinalysis suggest?
- What is the differential diagnosis for this disease?
- How do complement levels help in distinguishing causes of this disease?
- Which laboratory tests could help distinguish the cause of this process?

This patient's urinalysis contains protein, RBCs, and RBC casts, all highly suggestive of glomerular disease. Conditions leading to acute glomerulonephritis can generally be divided into diseases with a reduced complement level or those with normal complement levels. A scheme for delineating the differential diagnoses for acute glomerulonephritis is depicted in Table 45, along with the initial laboratory test or diagnostic procedure used to screen for each disease process.

TABLE 45. Glomerulonephritis

DISEASE	INITIAL DIAGNOSTIC TEST
Low serum complement states	
Systemic lupus erythematosus	ANA/dsDNA
Poststreptococcal glomerulonephritis	Antistreptolysin O (ASO) titer
Post-shunt nephritis	Shunt in place
Visceral abscess	Workup for abscess
Cryoglobulinemia	Serum cryos; HepB and HepC panels
Subacute bacterial endocarditis	Blood cultures; echocardiogram
Idiopathic membranoproliferative glomerulonephritis	Renal biopsy
Normal serum complement states	
IgA nephropathy	Renal biopsy
Henoch-Schönlein purpura (usually children)	Clinical diagnosis/renal biopsy if indicated
Goodpasture syndrome	Antiglomerular basement membrane Abs
Wegener's granulomatosis	cANCA (antineutrophilic cytoplasmic Abs)
Microscopic polyarteritis	pANCA positive

CASE CONTINUED

R.F. was admitted for fluid, electrolyte, and symptom management, as well as workup for her acute glomerulonephritis. The hospital nephrologist elected for supportive care rather than dialysis initially, so she received diuretics, antiemetics, electrolyte management, including exchange resins for the hyperkalemia, fluid restriction, and antihypertensive therapy as needed. A broad panel of laboratory tests was sent off as the nephrologists considered performing a renal biopsy. Laboratory tests returned as follows: ANA negative; HepBsAb, HepBcoreAb, and HepBsAg negative; HepC Ab negative; cryoglobulins negative; blood cultures × 2 negative; anti-GBM Ab negative; ASO titer 318 units/mL; cANCA and pANCA negative.

QUESTIONS

177. What is the most likely cause of this patient's glomerulonephritis?
    A. SLE
    B. IgA nephropathy
    C. Poststreptococcal GN
    D. Idiopathic membranoproliferative glomerulonephritis
    E. Acute tubular necrosis

178. The organism implicated in triggering poststreptococcal glomerulonephritis is:
    A. Group B *Streptococcus*
    B. *Streptococcus pneumoniae*
    C. *Streptococcus viridans*
    D. *Peptostreptococcus*
    E. Group A *Streptococcus*

179. The treatment for poststreptococcal glomerulonephritis is usually:
    A. Penicillin
    B. Steroids
    C. Cyclophosphamide
    D. Supportive care
    E. Renal transplant

180. IgA nephropathy is also known as:
    A. Polyarteritis nodosa
    B. Berger disease
    C. Gallavardin syndrome
    D. Thromboangiitis obliterans
    E. Kawasaki disease

CC/ID: 52-year-old man with a painful, swollen, hot right knee.

HPI: A.G. was awakened from sleep last night by exquisite pain in his right knee, which had become swollen and warm. He had felt well during the day preceding the onset of pain, and had attended a "crab-fest" that afternoon. He denies trauma to the joint, penetrating injuries, injections, or extramarital sexual contact. He lives in the city and does not enjoy hiking or camping, although he likes to fish. He cannot recall any tick exposures. He reports subjective fevers and sweats, but hasn't taken his temperature; the ROS is otherwise negative. Although no other joints currently hurt, he recalls an intensely painful left big toe several years ago that got better with "aspirin."

PMHx: Hypertension; binge EtOH; hernia repair. **Meds:** HCTZ, 25 mg PO QD **All:** NKDA

FHx/SHx: Parents both deceased; father had "arthritis." Married, with two adult children.

VS: Temp 39°C, BP 150/90, HR 100, RR 16, O_2 sat 98% RA

PE: *Gen:* large man, lying on gurney, nontoxic but uncomfortable. *HEENT:* unremarkable. *Neck:* supple, no thyromegaly or adenopathy. *Lungs:* clear. *CV:* RRR, normal S_1S_2, 2/6 HSM at apex. *Abdomen:* soft, NT/ND, +BS. *Ext:* no track marks; right knee swollen, warm, tender to touch; no swelling or lymphangitis; 2+ peripheral pulses. *Skin:* no rashes, no necrotic-appearing lesions. *GU:* no urethral discharge. *Neuro:* nonfocal.

Labs: WBC 13; Hct, Plt count normal; Cr 1.2; serum urate normal; INR 1.0.

THOUGHT QUESTIONS
- How would you summarize this patient's presentation?
- What is in your differential diagnosis?
- What diagnostic tests would you perform?

This 52-year-old man with a history significant for hypertension and alcohol use presents with the sudden onset of monoarthritis, fever, and mild leukocytosis. The differential diagnosis of an acute monoarthritis includes infectious arthritis (staphylococcal, streptococcal, gonococcal, *Borrelia burgdorferi*, HIV, occasionally TB or gram-negative rods), cellulitis, bursitis, trauma, and crystal deposition arthritis (gout and pseudogout).

Gout flares are usually characterized by the sudden onset of exquisitely painful monoarthritis (although an asymmetric polyarthritis is sometimes seen), commonly affecting the joints of the foot, ankle, or knee, and accompanied by fever and leukocytosis. The presenting symptoms are indistinguishable from those of infective arthritis, which can present simultaneously. It is therefore essential to perform arthrocentesis on any hot joint in order to distinguish between crystalline and septic arthritis. Joint fluid should be sent for WBC and differential, crystals, Gram stain, and culture. During a gout flare, the joint fluid is cloudy, with a WBC count of up to 50,000 cells/μL and 50% or more PMNs; the diagnosis is made by the presence of negatively birefringent, needle-shaped urate crystals when the fluid is examined under a polarizing microscope. In septic arthritis, the joint fluid WBC and predominance of PMNs are generally higher than those seen in gouty arthritis. In non-gonococcal septic arthritis, Gram stain and culture are usually positive. In gonococcal arthritis, however, Gram stain can be negative in 75% of cases, and culture in 50%. Identification of nontender, necrotic skin lesions characteristic of disseminated gonococcal infection, or pharyngeal, rectal, or urethral gonorrhea (often asymptomatic in disseminated disease) makes the diagnosis.

CASE CONTINUED

You aspirate 30 cc of thick, yellow, opaque fluid from the knee. The lab reports 25,000 WBC, 60% PMNs, no organisms on the Gram stain, and the presence of negatively birefringent, needle-like crystals.

QUESTIONS

181. You conclude that this patient:
     A. Has gout.
     B. Can't have gout, as the serum uric acid level is normal.
     C. Has gonococcal arthritis.
     D. Has acute osteoarthritis.

182. Which of the following measures would *not* be used to prevent this patient's condition from recurring:
     A. Dietary modification
     B. Changes in sexual practices
     C. Allopurinol
     D. Uricosuric agents

183. Treatment for an acute monoarthritis would never include:
     A. Ceftriaxone, 1 gram IV QD
     B. Nafcillin, 2 gram IV q6h; and gentamicin, 5.1 mg/kg IV QD
     C. Intra-articular or oral steroids, or oral NSAIDs
     D. Allopurinol
     E. Colchicine

184. If the laboratory technician had found positively birefringent, rhomboid crystals in the joint aspirate, your diagnosis would be:
     A. Gout
     B. Pseudogout
     C. Reiter syndrome
     D. A torn meniscus

CC/ID: 22-year-old woman presents with "sore wrist."

HPI: S.L. is a woman previously in good health, who presents to her primary care physician with complaints of left wrist pain. She is very active and sustained a minor basketball injury approximately 6 months ago to her right wrist, which resolved with rest and ice. However, S.L. has noticed swelling, warmth, and tenderness in her left wrist over the past 2 months without any known trauma to that area. She has tried ibuprofen, rest, ice, and elevation of the wrist without much alleviation of symptoms. She denies any numbness, tingling, or shooting pains in the region.

S.L. also admits to feeling generally fatigued over the past month and feeling uncharacteristically depressed without any clear life triggers. She complains of mild diffuse abdominal pain without any clear relation to food or bowel movements and has noticed occasional reddening of the skin on her face, which she attributes to sun exposure, and dry, itchy outer ears. Otherwise, she denies any other rashes, fevers, or chills, cough, SOB, nausea, vomiting, changes in bowel habits, blood in stool, urinary symptoms, vaginal discharge or menstrual irregularities (LMP 2 weeks ago), visual changes, or any other joint abnormalities. She has had no recent travel, camping, or exposure to woods, new medications, or animals.

PMHx: None **Meds:** None **All:** NKDA

SHx: No smoking, minimal EtOH, no drugs; patient is a lesbian with a monogamous partner; no h/o STDs and no h/o male partner. Works as office assistant, has never traveled outside of Bay Area.

FHx: Noncontributory. **VS:** Afebrile; BP 105/76; HR 62; RR 12; O_2 sat 99% on RA

PE: *Gen:* well-appearing young woman in NAD. *HEENT:* conjunctiva clear; OP clear; erythematous rash over nose and cheeks (Figure 47). *Neck:* No LAN. *CV:* RRR S_1S_2; no murmurs, gallops, or rubs. *Lungs:* CTA bilaterally. *Abdomen:* soft; +BS; NT/ND; no HSM. *Ext:* no edema; no rashes; left wrist with moderate effusion, mild warmth and tenderness to palpation; full ROM.

Labs: WBC 3.00 with normal differential; Hct 37.6; Plt 150,000. Lytes and LFTs WNL.

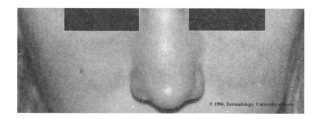

FIGURE 47 Erythematous plaques over nose and malar regions. (Copyrighted material is used with permission of the author, the University of Iowa and Virtual Hospital, www.vh.org.)

THOUGHT QUESTIONS

- Are there any unifying diagnoses for this patient's constellation of symptoms and lab findings?
- What is the best way to make the diagnosis?

This patient presents with left wrist effusion, warmth, and tenderness along with an erythematous rash over malar region, fatigue, depression, and leukopenia. Systemic processes that can lead to rashes, joint manifestations, and hematologic profile abnormalities include collagen vascular diseases and systemic infections (such as subacute bacterial endocarditis, disseminated gonococcal infections, and spirochetal infections such as syphilis or Lyme disease). Given this patient's age, gender, risk factors, and chronicity of global symptoms, a systemic autoimmune disease must be ruled out. Although most rheumatologic illnesses are diagnosed clinically, serologic testing can be useful. In addition, the patient should have a workup for infectious processes, including septic arthritis and systemic infections.

CASE CONTINUED

The patient's left wrist was aspirated and revealed a benign effusion; x-ray of the left wrist was normal. Three blood cultures were drawn and were negative. VDRL and FTA-ABS for syphilis were negative. UA was negative. ESR was 65. Serologic testing revealed a positive ANA and a positive anti-Smith antibody.

QUESTIONS

185. What is the most likely diagnosis of this patient's condition?
  A. Rheumatoid arthritis
  B. Sjögren syndrome
  C. Polyarteritis nodosa
  D. Systemic lupus erythematosus
  E. Polymyalgia rheumatica

186. Which of the following serologic tests is not included in the list of possible tests that can help diagnose this patient's syndrome?
  A. Anticardiolipin antibody
  B. Anti-centromere antibodies
  C. Anti-double-stranded-DNA antibody
  D. Anti-Smith antibodies
  E. False positive VDRL

187. Which of the following systems is *not* included in the 11 criteria of this condition established by the American Rheumatologic Association?
  A. Hematologic system
  B. Musculoskeletal system
  C. Gastrointestinal system
  D. Renal system
  E. Nervous system

188. How many criteria of the 11 mentioned above classifies a patient as having this diagnosis?
  A. 2
  B. 3
  C. 4
  D. 5
  E. 6

CASE 48 / SWOLLEN LEGS AND PUFFY EYELIDS IN A 35-YEAR-OLD WOMAN

CC/ID: 35-year-old woman complains of increasing fatigue and swelling.

HPI: N.S. was in her usual fair state of health until approximately 1 month ago, when her baseline fatigue began to increase. Over the next several weeks, her legs began to feel "heavy," and then "tight," and she noted progressive bilateral lower extremity swelling. Recently, her eyelids became "puffy." She came to the hospital because of the unremitting nature of her symptoms.

On ROS, she notes night sweats and gradual weight loss over the past 6 months. She denies headaches, swollen lymph nodes, cough, SOB, abdominal pain, nausea, vomiting, or diarrhea. She has not noticed any bleeding other than during menstruation.

PMHx: Community-acquired pneumonia 1 and 3 years ago, treated as an outpatient. Recurrent candidal vulvovaginitis, treated with oral fluconazole. ASCUS on last Pap smear; did not keep follow-up appointment for repeat exam.

Meds: None   **All:** NKDA

SHx: Estranged from her husband. Has two healthy teenage children. Works in retail. No cigarettes, EtOH, or illicit substances.

FHx: Father, sister with sickle cell trait.   **VS:** Temp 97.4°F, BP 138/80, HR 80, RR 16, O_2 sat 98% on RA

PE: *Gen:* thin, with engorged eyelids, appears chronically ill. *HEENT:* as above; OP without lesions or thrush. *Neck:* supple; no adenopathy; 2+ carotid upstrokes; JVP 12 cm above midaxilla. *Lungs:* CTA. *CV:* RRR; normal S_1S_2; no murmurs. *Abdomen:* soft, NT/ND; +BS; no HSM. *Ext:* 2+ pitting edema to just below the knee bilaterally; no cords or erythema. *Neuro:* nonfocal.

Labs: Chemistries normal except for BUN 20; Cr 1.7. Heme: WBC 4.1; Hgb 11.5; Hct 36; Plt 220,000. UA: 4+ protein; sediment normal. *CXR:* no infiltrates, edema, cardiomegaly, or vertebral abnormalities.

THOUGHT QUESTIONS

- How would you summarize this patient's presentation?
- What tests would help you determine the cause of her edema?

This 35-year-old woman presents with progressive peripheral edema developing over the last month, accompanied by mild renal insufficiency, leukopenia, borderline anemia, and marked proteinuria, and with a past medical history notable for infections.

The differential diagnosis of lower extremity edema includes right-sided heart failure; end-stage liver disease with portal hypertension; bilateral DVTs below the bifurcation of the iliac veins, or venous thrombus in the inferior vena cava or above; external compression of the venous return from the lower extremities, such as tumors of the GI or reproductive tract; lymphedema; myxedema; or the nephrotic syndrome. The development of eyelid edema suggests a systemic process, rather than obstruction of venous return from the lower extremities. In addition, the finding of proteinuria on urine dipstick is suspicious for nephrotic syndrome, and should be investigated further with a 24-hour urine protein collection. The serum albumin should be determined as well; as the urine dipstick test detects only albumin, however, the presence of abnormal paraproteins in the urinary sediment should be sought with the sulfosalicylic acid test. In the meantime, it would be reasonable to check liver enzymes, bilirubin, and alkaline phosphatase, as well as serologies for viral hepatitis. Testing for less common causes of liver disease and hypothyroidism can wait until nephrotic syndrome is ruled out, as can imaging studies to look for thrombi, and echocardiography to assess cardiac function.

CASE CONTINUED

The 24-hour urine collection yields 4.3 grams of protein. The serum albumin is 2.1 g/dL. Hepatic enzymes, serum bilirubin, and alkaline phosphatase are normal, as are the PT and PTT. The patient is HCV-antibody neg, HBV sAg neg, HBV sAb pos, HBV core antibody pos.

QUESTIONS

189. This patient's edema is most likely caused by:
    A. Chronic liver disease
    B. Nephrotic syndrome
    C. Unclear; would order a transthoracic echocardiogram
    D. Unclear; would order an abdominal CT scan

190. Based on your answer to Question 189, which of the following additional tests would you order?
    A. Liver biopsy
    B. Renal biopsy
    C. HIV serology
    D. (B) and (C)
    E. (A), (B), and (C)

191. Suppose that the patient is HIV-infected. Therapeutic options include:
    A. Steroids
    B. Cyclophosphamide
    C. Highly active antiretroviral therapy
    D. (A) and (C)
    E. (A), (B), and (C)

192. Depending on additional lab tests, you might want to consider adding any of the following *except*:
    A. A loop diuretic
    B. An ACE inhibitor
    C. Intravenous albumin supplementation
    D. Coumadin
    E. An HMG-CoA-reductase-inhibitor

CC/ID: 51-year-old woman presents with persistent right elbow pain.

HPI: R.A. presents to her primary care physician with complaints of right elbow pain. She has a h/o chronic fatigue syndrome and comes to primary MD frequently with requests for further diagnostic workup into her condition. She is on a waiting list for a Chronic Fatigue Syndrome clinic and takes various herbal preparations, obtains acupuncture once a week, and maintains special diets. She also is physically active, jogging twice a week, and playing tennis once a week. Over the past 4 months, R.A. has noted increased pain in her right elbow with swelling over the joint. She also complains of reduced ROM and stiffness in the elbow and both wrists, which usually improve throughout the day with activity. She notes that chronic fatigue has been worsening over this time period, despite sleeping 14 hours a day, and feels generally weak. She reports low-grade subjective fevers for about 2 months. She denies night sweats, weight loss, abdominal pain, nausea, vomiting, cough, SOB, or bowel or urinary symptoms, but complains of dry eyes and mouth, which she attributes to St. John's wort. She has no other joint problems or rashes. She is worried that she is "coming down with fibromyalgia."

PMHx: Total abdominal hysterectomy 15 years previously, h/o depression and anxiety.

Meds: Various herbal preparations for chronic fatigue, including Enada (absorbable form of the coenzyme NADH) and St. John's wort.

All: NKDA

SHx: No smoking; no EtOH; no illicit drugs; lives alone with 4 cats—no recent scratches or bites.

FHx: Mother had Sjögren syndrome. **VS:** Temp 37.9°C, BP 142/90, HR 85, RR 12

PE: *Gen:* anxious-appearing female in NAD. *HEENT:* mild conjunctival injections bilaterally; OP clear. *Neck:* no LAN. *CV:* RRR, S_1S_2; no murmurs or gallops but faint rub audible, increased with inspiration. *Lungs:* CTA bilaterally. *Abdomen:* soft; obese; +BS; NT/ND; no HSM. *Ext:* mild swelling of the wrist joints bilaterally R>L without tenderness, warmth, or erythema; right olecranon with a palpable effusion, tenderness to touch and pain with flexion/extension, moderately warm with reddish-blue discoloration over the joint; no other joint abnormalities; no rashes; no pain with palpation in the muscles of the posterior neck or back.

Labs: WBC 9.60; Hct 34.0; Plt 200K; lytes, LFTs, and fasting glucose all WNL.

THOUGHT QUESTIONS
- What is the differential diagnosis of this patient's condition?
- Which lab test(s) should be sent next?

This patient has an inflamed elbow joint, with warmth, tenderness to palpation, limited ROM, and erythema. The differential diagnosis of an inflamed joint is shown in Table 49.

TABLE 49. Causes of Arthritis
Infectious processes
Bacterial arthritis (most commonly, *Staphylococcus aureus*, streptococcal species, *Neisseria gonorrhoeae*)
Viral arthritis (including rubella, hepatitis B, parvovirus)
Fungal arthritis
Immune-mediated processes
Reiter's syndrome (reactive arthritis)
Autoimmune processes (including psoriatic arthritis, rheumatoid arthritis, systemic lupus erythematosus, Sjögren syndrome, systemic sclerosis, polymyalgia rheumatica, other vasculitides, inflammatory bowel disease)
Acute rheumatic fever
Crystal-mediated processes
Gout and calcium pyrophosphate disease (pseudogout)
Other
Erosive osteoarthritis
Sarcoidosis
Amyloidosis
Paraneoplastic syndrome

Given the destructive implications of septic arthritis, joint aspiration should be the first procedure performed to rule out infection in the joint space. The fluid should be sent for cell count with differential, chemistries, Gram stain, and culture.

CASE CONTINUED

The patient's right elbow was aspirated to reveal a yellow, moderately viscous, cloudy fluid. White blood cell count was 10,000 with 62% polymorphonuclear leukocytes. Glucose level was 80 (peripheral glucose 100), total protein was 4.0 g/dL. Gram stain and cultures were negative. Peripheral ESR was 117; serum RF was positive.

QUESTIONS

193. The most likely diagnosis in this case is:
    A. Septic arthritis
    B. Rheumatoid arthritis
    C. Psoriatic arthritis
    D. Fibromyalgia
    E. Gout

194. Which HLA allele is most frequently associated with RA in Caucasians?
    A. HLA-B27
    B. HLA-B28
    C. HLA-DR2
    D. HLA-DR3
    E. HLA-DR4

195. What percentage of patients with rheumatoid arthritis are positive for rheumatoid factor?
    A. 10%
    B. 20%
    C. 50%
    D. 80%
    E. 100%

196. Which of the following would *not* be considered as initial therapy for this patient with rheumatoid arthritis?
    A. NSAIDs
    B. Methotrexate
    C. Plaquenil
    D. Cyclosporine
    E. Prednisone

CASE 50 / TIRED OF UREMIA

CC/ID: 73-year-old man with a h/o hypertension, diabetes mellitus, and ESRD presents with SOB.

HPI: H.D. has a long h/o hypertension, poorly controlled diabetes mellitus, end-stage renal disease, and on hemodialysis for the past 7 years. He underwent a cadaveric renal transplant 5 years ago and was off dialysis for approximately 2 months, but rejected the renal transplant, necessitating reinstitution of hemodialysis. Since then, H.D. has been on the waiting list for a second cadaveric renal transplant, with multiple complications of his renal failure, including bleeding, repeated failure of his AV fistula grafts, nausea, weakness, fatigue, and malnutrition. H.D.'s hypertension has been extremely difficult to control, and he has severe inoperable three-vessel coronary artery disease with frequent angina. H.D. has missed multiple hemodialysis sessions in the past month and presents to his physician with SOB and signs of fluid overload. He comes to discuss discontinuation of his hemodialysis sessions. He states, "Doc, I'm in my right mind and this is no way to live. I'm going to stop anyway; I just want your blessing."

PMHx: ESRD as above. Carotid artery stenosis. Type II DM for 15 years, poorly controlled. DVT 3 years ago. Hypertension for 25 years. Depression. Severe coronary artery disease after NQWMI 10 years ago. Benign prostatic hypertrophy. Peripheral vascular disease—claudication with 2 blocks of walking. Hyperlipidemia.

Meds:

1. Lisinopril, 5 mg PO QD;
2. Amlodipine, 10 mg PO QD;
3. Clonidine, 0.3 mg patch each week;
4. Hydralazine, 25 mg PO QID;
5. Prazosin, 10 mg PO BID;
6. Nitroglycerin PRN;
7. ECASA, 325 mg PO QD;
8. Simvastatin, 20 mg PO QD;
9. Prozac, 20 mg PO QD;
10. Insulin scale

All: NKDA

SHx: Has smoked one-half ppd for 50 years; no EtOH or drugs; widower with three children.

VS: Temp 36.8°C, BP 170/115, HR 100, RR 16, O_2 sat 93% RA

PE: *Gen:* chronically ill elderly man in mild respiratory distress. *HEENT:* cataracts; TMs clear; OP clear *Neck:* JVD elevated to ~10 cm; no LAN. *CV:* RRR S_1S_2; S_3S_4 gallops present; faint rub heard on inspiration; no murmurs. *Lungs:* crackles halfway up bilaterally. *Abdomen:* soft; +BS; NT/ND; no HSM; healed surgical scar from renal transplant. *Ext:* 2+ edema halfway up to knees; multiple ecchymoses over lower extremities; sites of former AV graft fistulas visible but no erythema, tenderness, warmth; current AV fistula with bruit auscultated and thrill to palpation present.

Labs: Last laboratory values available: Na 131; K 5.8; Cl 110; HCO_3 15; BUN 65; Cr 5.6; Ca 6.8; Phos 6.2; WBC 6.4; Hct 30.8

THOUGHT QUESTIONS
- What is the prognosis of patients with ESRD on hemodialysis without renal transplant?
- What are the main causes of ESRD in the U.S.?

The annual mortality rate for hemodialysis patients is approximately 20% to 25%, an estimate that does not include the additional mortality imposed by the comorbid condition of diabetes mellitus. Patients with ESRD and diabetes on hemodialysis can have an annual mortality of up to 40%. Cardiovascular disease accounts for most cases of mortality in patients with ESRD on hemodialysis.

TABLE 50. Causes of Chronic Renal Failure

DISEASE	PERCENTAGE OF CASES
Diabetes	37.0
Type I	15.0
Type II	22.0
Hypertension (includes renal artery stenosis)	29.0
Glomerulonephritis	11.0
Tubulointerstitial disease (includes obstruction)	4.5
Polycystic kidney disease	3.5
Secondary glomerulonephritis (includes vasculitis)	2.4
Neoplasms (includes multiple myeloma)	1.6
HIV nephropathy	1.0
Miscellaneous/unknown	5.0–10.0

The most common cause of chronic renal failure in the U.S. is diabetes mellitus, accounting for almost 40% of all causes of renal failure (Table 50). Between 20% and 40% of patients with type I diabetes develop renal damage. There is a lower prevalence of kidney damage with type II diabetes, because many patients develop type II diabetes at a later age and die prematurely from cardiovascular disease before renal failure develops. However, more patients with chronic renal failure have type II diabetes than type I, because many more patients with diabetes have type II disease. Hypertension is recorded as the second most common cause of chronic renal failure, but confounding may occur as renal failure of any origin will usually result in hypertension. Various forms of glomerulonephritis, such as idiopathic membranous nephropathy, IgA nephropathy, and lupus nephritis, make up the third most common cause of renal failure. Together, diabetes, hypertension, and glomerulonephritis are responsible for nearly 80% of cases of chronic renal failure. Numerous other diseases as listed in Table 50 make up the remaining causes of renal failure. The cause is categorized as unknown in approximately 5% to 10% of cases.

CASE CONTINUED

After numerous discussions between H.D., his family, his primary care physician, his nephrologist, and the social worker in the dialysis center, agreement was reached that the patient was competent to make his own decisions and dictate the course of his care. The patient was continued on antihypertensives, calcium and vitamin D supplementation, and phosphate-binding therapy, and was provided with bicarbonate supplementation at home. The patient stopped attending his hemodialysis sessions and died peacefully a week later in his son's home.

QUESTIONS

197. Which of the following antihypertensives have been shown to slow the progression of several types of renal failure, including diabetic nephropathy?
A. Beta blockers
B. Thiazide diuretics
C. Hydralazine
D. ACE inhibitors
E. Nitrates

198. Which drug class should be used as second-line antihypertensive therapy for hypertension in diabetic nephropathy in terms of slowing progression to renal failure? (First-line therapy is answer to Question 1.)
A. Hydralazine
B. Beta blockers
C. Calcium channel blockers
D. Thiazide diuretics
E. Nitrates

199. The anemia of chronic renal failure is due primarily to:
A. Iron deficiency
B. Low erythropoietin levels
C. Hemolysis
D. Blood loss from dialysis
E. Splenic sequestration

200. The kidney is important in the regulation of calcium homeostasis through its production of the following hormone:
A. Calcitriol
B. Parathyroid hormone (PTH)
C. Calcitonin
D. Phosphorus
E. 22-oxacalcitriol

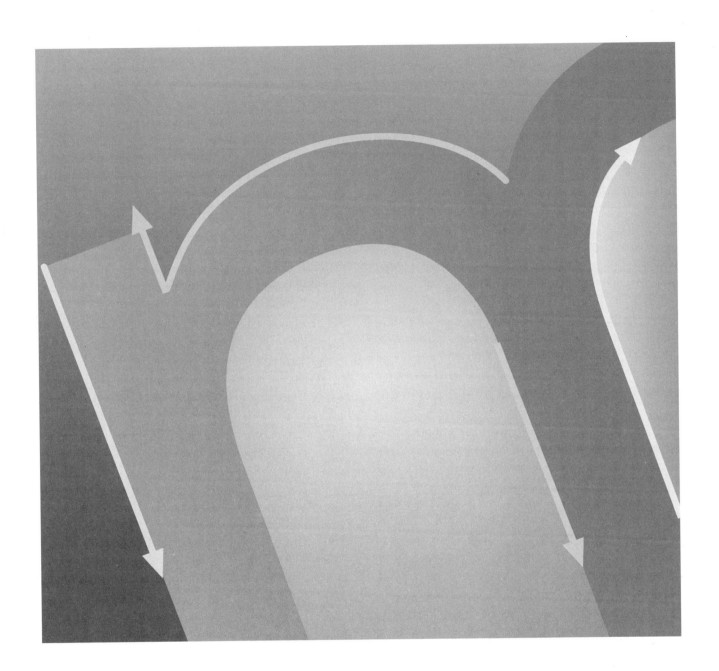

ANSWERS

CASE PRESENTATIONS

CASES PRESENTING WITH SHORTNESS OF BREATH
Case 1. Acute Shortness of Breath in a Young Woman
Case 2. Very Short of Breath
Case 3. Shortness of Breath Over One Year
Case 4. Chronic Shortness of Breath
Case 5. Hypertensive, Short of Breath, and Dizzy
Case 6. Fever and Shortness of Breath
Case 7. Young Woman with Shortness of Breath
Case 8. White Lungs
Case 9. Fever, Sweats, and Painful Cough in an Exotic Dancer
Case 10. Fever, Productive Cough, Shortness of Breath
Case 11. Shortness of Breath and Palpitations

CASES PRESENTING WITH PAIN IN AND AROUND THE CHEST
Case 12. Chest Pain, Shortness of Breath
Case 13. Severe Back Pain
Case 14. Syncopal Episode
Case 15. 49-Year-Old Man with Left Shoulder Pain
Case 16. 53-Year-Old Man with Chest Pain

CASES PRESENTING WITH PAIN IN AND AROUND THE ABDOMEN
Case 17. Eating French Fries Hurts!
Case 18. Tarry, Smelly Stools and Hematemesis
Case 19. Fever, Right Upper Quadrant Pain
Case 20. Diarrhea on the Plane
Case 21. Fever, Diarrhea, and Abdominal Cramping in a Young Man
Case 22. 41-Year-Old Man with Abdominal Pain
Case 23. Hurts to Eat
Case 24. Gnawing Epigastric Pain, Nausea, and Vomiting
Case 25. Too Much Tylenol
Case 26. Fever, Swollen Abdomen, Drowsy, and Yellow
Case 27. Fever, Abdominal Pain, and Foot Drop

CASES PRESENTING WITH A HORMONAL BALANCE
Case 28. Young Woman, Breathing Hard, with Sunken Cheeks
Case 29. Slowing Down
Case 30. Cancerous Calcification
Case 31. Dizzy When I Stand Up
Case 32. Keeping That Sugar Down
Case 33. Jittery

CASES PRESENTING WITH PATIENTS WANTING TO KEEP IN GOOD HEALTH
Case 34. 65-Year-Old Woman Who Hasn't Seen a Doctor Recently
Case 35. Calculating Cholesterol
Case 36. Reaction to TB

CASES PRESENTING WITH PAIN IN AND AROUND THE HEAD
Case 37. Headache, Fever
Case 38. Stuffy Nose
Case 39. Fever, Sore Throat

CASES PRESENTING WITH TROUBLE IN THE BLOOD
Case 40. Bleeding Gums
Case 41. 50-Year-Old Man with Fatigue and Nosebleed
Case 42. Abnormal Lab Values in a Man with an Abscess
Case 43. Feverish, Bleeding, and Confused
Case 44. New Relationship

CASES PRESENTING WITH SWELLING
Case 45. Swollen After a Sore Throat
Case 46. Painful, Swollen Knee
Case 47. Sore Wrist
Case 48. Swollen Legs, Puffy Eyelids in a 35-Year-Old Woman
Case 49. Swollen, and Painful Joints
Case 50. Tired of Uremia

DIAGNOSIS

Pulmonary Embolus
Asthma
Primary Pulmonary Hypertension
COPD (Chronic Obstructive Pulmonary Disease)
Hypertensive Emergency
Empyema
Cardiomyopathy with Congestive Heart Failure
Amiodarone-Induced Pulmonary Fibrosis
Infections in IV Drug Users
Community-Acquired Pneumonia
Atrial Fibrillation

Unstable Angina
Aortic Dissection
Aortic Stenosis
Myocardial Infarction
Non-Cardiac Chest Pain

Gastroesophageal Reflux Disease
Gastrointestinal Bleed
Cholecystitis and Cholangitis
Traveler's Diarrhea
Inflammatory Bowel Disease
Ischemic Bowel
Candidal Esophagitis
Acute Pancreatitis
Fulminant Hepatic Failure
End Stage Liver Disease
Vasculitis/Polyarteritis Nodosa

Diabetic Ketoacidosis
Hypothyroidism
Hypercalcemia
Adrenal Insufficiency
Chronic Diabetes Mellitus
Hyperthyroidism

Adult Screening
Hypercholesterolemia
Reaction to PPD

Bacterial Meningitis
Sinusitis
Pharyngitits

Idiopathic Thrombocytopenic Purpura (ITP)
Acute Leukemia
Anemia
Thrombotic Thrombocytopenic Purpura (TTP)
Acute HIV Infection

Acute Renal Failure
Gout
Systemic Lupus Erythematosus (SLE)
Nephrotic Syndrome
Rheumatoid Arthritis
Chronic Renal Failure

1–C

The ventilation-perfusion scan remains the most common diagnostic test used when pulmonary embolism is suspected: Perfusion defects and ventilation-perfusion mismatches indicate possible areas of clot. The Prospective Investigation of Pulmonary Embolism Diagnosis (PIOPED) study data showed that, to provide adequate data for diagnosis, lung scan results must be combined with clinical suspicion for a pulmonary embolus. Spiral (helical) CT with contrast is an increasingly popular diagnostic technique for acute pulmonary embolus; this modality is better suited for central emboli, as peripheral visualization of the upper and lower lobes is limited. MRI has excellent sensitivity and specificity for pulmonary embolism but has potential inconveniences for studying critically ill patients. Pulmonary arteriography has remained the gold standard technique for the diagnosis of acute pulmonary embolism, with excellent specificity and sensitivity, although its safety issues and difficulty limit its use. Measurement of circulating D-dimer by ELISA has excellent sensitivity (but not specificity) for the diagnosis of pulmonary embolus; a normal level can rule out thrombotic disease, but an elevated level is not specific for thrombosis.

2–D

In acute pulmonary embolus, ECG findings are present in the majority of patients and include nonspecific T wave changes, ST segment abnormalities, and axis deviation. Only one-third of patients with massive or submassive emboli have manifestations of acute right heart strain (cor pulmonale), which include right bundle branch block, large P waves (P-wave pulmonale), right axis deviation, or the classic $S_1Q_3T_3$ pattern (a prominent S wave in lead I and a Q wave with an inverted T wave in lead III). Patients can also have normal ECGs in the presence of acute pulmonary embolus. Peaked T waves are usually a feature of hyperkalemia or myocardial damage.

3–B

Trousseau's syndrome is characterized by migratory superficial thrombophlebitis of the upper or lower extremities and is strongly linked to cancer. The cause of Trousseau's syndrome is uncertain, but this hypercoagulable state seems to be induced by release of a tissue thromboplastin from malignant cells, which ultimately initiates the extrinsic coagulation pathway.

TABLE A3. Main Risk Factors for Thrombotic Syndromes

Primary hypercoagulable states
Antithrombin III/Heparin disorders: Antithrombin deficiency, heparin cofactor II deficiency
Protein C/Protein S disorders: Protein C deficiency, protein S deficiency, activated protein C resistance, factor V Leiden, thrombomodulin dysfunction
Prothrombin gene mutation
Fibrinolytic disorders: Hypoplasminogenemia, dysplasminogenemia, plasminogen activator deficiency, dysfibrinogenemia
Hyperhomocystinemia: Cystathionine beta-synthetase deficiency, remethylation pathway defects, acquired hyperhomocystinemia (pyridoxine, cobalamin, folate deficiency)

Secondary hypercoagulable states
Malignancy (Trousseau syndrome)
Disseminated intravascular coagulation (DIC)
Myeloproliferative disorders and paroxysmal nocturnal hemoglobinuria
Antiphospholipid antibody syndrome
Pregnancy
Oral contraceptives, especially when combined with smoking in patients >35 years of age
Postoperative states
Trauma
Prolonged immobility
Congestive heart failure (usually secondary to immobility)
Nephrotic syndrome, ESRD

4–E

Unfractionated heparin and hirudin increase the PTT, which should be monitored during therapy for efficacy and safety. Coumadin is the trade name for warfarin; this anticoagulant affects the PT. The international normalized ratio (INR) standardizes the PT measurements from each laboratory and is used to determine the optimum dose of warfarin. Low-molecular-weight heparin (LMWH) has recently been demonstrated to be efficacious and safe in the treatment of acute DVT/pulmonary embolism and can be administered subcutaneously once or twice a day without monitoring the PTT.

5–D

Respiratory alkalosis leads to hypokalemia, as [K+] ions rush out of cells to compensate for the relative paucity of [H+] ions in the face of increased CO_2 elimination; however, this patient has respiratory acidosis, not alkalosis. The most likely explanation for his hypokalemia at this point is that administration of β-agonists leads to a transcellular inward shift of potassium through the Na+/K+-ATPase pump; this effect can reduce serum K+ 0.5–1.0 mEq/L within 30 minutes after administration and be sustained for at least 2 hours.

6–B

Systemic steroids should be administered to reduce the inflammatory component of this

ANSWERS

patient's acute asthma exacerbation. Studies have shown equal efficacy in steroid treatment administered orally or intravenously. Given the patient's mechanical ventilation status, Solu-Medrol, 40–60 mg IV q6h, will most likely be administered and then switched to PO prednisone once oral intake is feasible.

7–A

Though rare, pneumothorax and pneumomediastinum are complications of mechanical ventilation, given the positive end-expiratory pressure. Breaching of the normal laryngeal and mucosal barriers to infection with the endotracheal tube, along with colonization by multiple organisms, predisposes a ventilated patient to pneumonia. Tracheomalacia can occur after prolonged intubation, although soft balloons have decreased this problem. Pulmonary hypertension is not an immediate problem associated with mechanical ventilation.

8–E

The alveolar-arterial O_2 gradient equation is:

$$\text{A-a gradient} = 714 \times F_{IO_2} - 1.25\,(pCO_2) - pO_2$$
$$\text{At room air, } F_{IO_2} = 0.21$$

so

$$\text{A-a gradient} = 150 - 1.25\,(pCO_2) - pO_2$$
$$= 150 - 1.25\,(59) - 74 = 2.25\,(<5)$$

9–D, 10–A, 11–E, 12–E

It is very likely that this patient has primary pulmonary hypertension, because the workup rules out the most common sources of secondary pulmonary hypertension. Right heart catheterization is required to determine the hemodynamic severity of the disease, as well as to rule out an intracardiac shunt. Primary pulmonary hypertension is a rare, irreversible disease with a generally poor prognosis. It is therefore essential to rule out reversible or removable causes of secondary pulmonary hypertension when a patient presents with signs of right heart failure.

Because patients with primary pulmonary hypertension depend on systemic blood pressure to maintain perfusion of the right ventricle, sudden decreases in systemic blood pressure can precipitate right heart ischemia and death. Careful use of diuretics can alleviate dyspnea and peripheral edema. Vasodilators, such as calcium channel blockers and intravenous prostacyclin, have been shown to reduce symptoms and improve mortality in some patients with primary pulmonary hypertension, but identification of these patients should be done using short-acting vasodilators during the close hemodynamic monitoring allowed by right-sided cardiac catheterization. In addition, some authorities recommend chronic anticoagulation even in the absence of angiographic evidence of thromboembolic disease, because microthrombi may be difficult to detect.

Demonstration of chronic thromboembolic disease changes the diagnosis to secondary pulmonary hypertension, and requires anticoagulation and workup for causes of hypercoagulability. This would include factor V Leiden; antithrombin III, protein C, and protein S deficiencies; the presence of anticardiolipin antibody or lupus anticoagulant; ulcerative colitis; dysfibrinogenemia, or abnormal plasminogen; heparin-induced thrombocytopenia; and possibly certain occult cancers (lung, pancreas, breast, ovarian, GI, GU, lymphoma, or brain).

13–C

The only genetic risk factor for emphysema known to date is a hereditary deficiency of α_1-antitrypsin, a major circulating inhibitor of serine proteases. Individuals with α_1-antitrypsin deficiency have at least a 20-fold increased risk of developing emphysema, with 80% to 90% of deficient individuals eventually developing this condition. α_1-antitrypsin deficiency is especially dangerous for smokers, in whom it is associated with the accelerated development of emphysema and premature mortality.

14–E

Ipratopium bromide (Atrovent) is an anticholinergic medication that blocks the effects of acetylcholine on a variety of muscarinic receptor types: most important in the pathophysiology of COPD are the M3 receptors at the motor end plate. Short-acting inhaled anticholinergics have a bronchodilating effect that generally lasts longer than that of short-acting β_2-agonists. However, the decision to use inhaled β_2-agonists, anticholinergic agents, or a combination of both, is dictated by the individual response of the patient.

15–D

Smoking cessation is effective in reducing the severity of COPD at any stage of disease, although its main efficacy lies in the earlier stages.

16–B

COPD is the fourth leading cause of death worldwide. The ranking of causes of death worldwide is

1. Heart disease
2. Cerebrovascular disease
3. Accidents
4. COPD
5. Pneumonia and influenza
6. Diabetes mellitus
7. Suicide
8. HIV infection

17–D, 18–B, 19–E

In treating hypertensive *emergency*, the goal is a prompt, partial decrease in blood pressure that prevents end-organ damage, without dropping the blood pressure so low as to risk neurologic, coronary, or renal ischemia. Initially reducing the MAP by no more than 25%, or reducing the diastolic blood pressure by one-third are two commonly used methods; the former comes from the Sixth Report of the Joint National Committee on Detection, Evaluation And Treatment of High Blood Pressure (JNC VI). Calculating the MAP is a little more complicated than simply averaging the systolic and diastolic pressures. The actual calculation is the result of a weighted average, as most patients will be in diastole approximately twice as long as systole. However, determining a target MAP rarely involves much back-calculating, as most blood pressure machines used in hospitals track the MAP with each blood pressure measurement.

Intravenous sodium nitroprusside, nitroglycerin, and labetalol are three titratable, effective, and short-acting agents used in the treatment of hypertensive emergency. Nitroprusside is the most potent and rapid agent; its use requires placement of an arterial line for continuous blood pressure monitoring. IV nitroglycerin can also be titrated, but is somewhat less effective than nitroprusside, and runs the risk of inducing (temporary) tolerance and thus loss of effectiveness. Labetalol is longer acting and less easy to titrate, but does not cause wide swings in pressure. Nitroglycerin and labetalol are particularly useful in treating concomitant cardiac ischemia.

Many other agents have been used to control hypertensive emergencies: esmolol, a short-acting beta-blocker; enalaprilat, an intravenous version of the ACE inhibitor enalapril; diazoxide; and hydralazine. Sublingual nifedipine causes drastic swings in blood pressure, as well as reflex tachycardia, and does not have a role in the treatment of hypertensive emergency. Additionally, it has been associated with increased mortality when used in patients who have cardiac ischemia.

20–A

The diagnosis of hypertensive *urgency* is given to patients who present with highly elevated blood pressure, even with optic disc edema, but no evidence of end-organ damage. The goal of therapy is to partially reduce blood pressure, which is usually achieved with oral medications. It is important to rule out end-organ damage with appropriate testing.

21–E

The pleural fluid LDH/serum LDH >0.60 indicates a transudate; the pH <7.3, high WBC count consisting of PMNs, the Gram stain, and history all suggest empyema. Proper treatment includes culture-directed antibiotics and urgent, thorough drainage through a chest tube. There are several reasons for drainage: to evacuate infected material, and to avoid the formation of a fibrinous peel, which can lead to lung trapping and a nonfunctioning lung. An empyema detected in the early, free-flowing stage can be treated with tube drainage and antibiotics. Once loculations develop, instillation of thrombolytics through the chest tube can be attempted, but many patients will eventually require open or thoracoscopic decortication of the pleural peel.

22–C

This patient's empyema developed from a parapneumonic effusion caused by an undiagnosed bacterial pneumonia. Had the physician who ordered the chest x-ray 2 weeks earlier remembered to look at the film, the pneumonia could have been treated with antibiotics alone. The moral of the story is to check the results of the tests you order.

23–B

Not all effusions require therapeutic or even diagnostic thoracentesis. In a patient with known CHF and effusions that do not cause respiratory distress, and who has no other reason to have effusions besides a CHF exacerbation, the effusions should resolve with treatment for heart failure. If there is any doubt as to the cause of the effusions, or should the effusions result in dyspnea, then thoracentesis should be performed.

ANSWERS

24–A

A small pneumothorax, defined as less than 15% of the hemithorax on chest radiogram, will usually resorb spontaneously. This can be hastened by placing the patient on 100% O_2 by face mask. Serial chest radiograms are important to monitor the progress of reexpansion.

25–C, 26–D, 27–E, 28–B

This patient is presenting in CHF, with dyspnea, tachypnea, elevated jugular venous pressure, an S_3, and bilateral crackles on examination, as well as decreased room air oxygen saturation and interstitial infiltrates in a pattern classic for pulmonary edema on chest x-ray. Loop diuretics, IV morphine, and nitrates relieve acute pulmonary edema by decreasing left ventricular preload. In addition, low-dose morphine reduces the anxiety of dyspnea; higher doses may depress ventilatory drive and should be avoided. Supplemental oxygen relieves dyspnea while you wait for other agents to work. Although beta-blockers have a place in the long-term treatment of CHF, they are not used in the acute setting. The patient in cardiogenic shock may require endotracheal intubation and mechanical ventilation, and intravenous positive inotropic agents.

The cardiomyopathies fall into three broad categories: dilated, hypertrophic, and restrictive/constrictive. Echocardiography is very useful in distinguishing among them, although cardiac catheterization is sometimes necessary as well. Characterized by left ventricular dilatation and dysfunction on echocardiogram, and high diastolic pressures and low cardiac output on catheterization, dilated cardiomyopathy has many causes: ischemic damage; idiopathic causes; chronic effects of hypertension or valvular disease; viral myocarditis; alcohol use; hyper- or hypothyroidism; the peripartum state; and drug toxicities, particularly doxorubicin. An echocardiogram showing left ventricular hypertrophy, normal to increased cardiac function, and diastolic dysfunction would suggest hypertrophic cardiomyopathy, which can be caused by a genetic mutation or by chronic hypertension. Finding normal to slightly reduced ventricular volumes and function and thickened walls on echocardiography, as well as increased bilateral diastolic filling pressures on catheterization, suggests constrictive or restrictive disease. Pericarditis, surgery, or radiation can cause constrictive cardiomyopathy. Endomyocardial fibrosis, Loeffler's endocarditis, and infiltrative diseases such as amyloidosis, hemochromatosis, and sarcoidosis cause restrictive cardiomyopathy. Differentiating constrictive from restrictive cardiomyopathy is difficult but important, as constrictive cardiomyopathy can be reversed with pericardial stripping. The finding of pericardial thickening on CT or MRI scan argues for constrictive disease, whereas the finding of infiltrative disease on endomyocardial biopsy argues for restrictive disease.

The treatment of heart failure depends on the type of underlying cardiomyopathy. The diastolic dysfunction of hypertrophic cardiomyopathy often responds to the calcium channel blockers verapamil or diltiazem, or to beta-blockers. Cardiomyopathy caused by endocrinopathies, alcohol use, a constrictive process, or certain kinds of ischemia (so-called "hibernating myocardium") may improve with treatment of the underlying condition. Based on her examination and echocardiogram, patient A.M. has CHF due to dilated cardiomyopathy. The clinical history of a respiratory tract infection preceding the onset of her symptoms suggests a viral myocarditis. Some experts would proceed with endomyocardial biopsy and, if an acute inflammatory infiltrate is found, immunosuppressive therapy; this is, however an area of controversy.

Medications used to treat any patient with dilated cardiomyopathy, or left ventricular systolic dysfunction, include: *thiazide* or *loop diuretics*; *ACE inhibitors, spironolactone, beta-blockers,* and *digoxin*. Both diuretics and ACE inhibitors decrease cardiac workload by decreasing left ventricular preload; ACE inhibitors also decrease afterload through arterial vasodilation. Beta-blockers may reduce ongoing myocardial damage and arrhythmias by blocking chronic catecholamine stimulation. ACE inhibitors, spironolactone, and beta blockers have all been shown to reduce mortality in patients with CHF, depending on the degree of disease. Digoxin reduces the symptoms of CHF with no overall mortality benefit; it decreases mortality due to cardiac failure, while increasing mortality due to ischemia and arrhythmia. The use of oral inotropic agents other than digoxin has been shown to increase mortality in clinical trials. Finally, some experts advocate the use of anticoagulation in patients with CHF and very low cardiac output (<20%), who are prone to the development of intracardiac thrombi.

29–D

The chest x-ray shows a diffuse interstitial reticulonodular process most prominent in the lower lobes, suggestive of a diffuse interstitial process of unclear cause. The PFTs show a restrictive pattern and a reduced diffusing capacity, also suggestive of interstitial lung disease. The echocardiogram showing relatively intact LV function argues against CHF as a cause of this condition. And finally, the high-resolution CT showing the asymmetric lung opacities with the ground-glass appearance is also consistent with interstitial lung disease.

30–C

Interstitial lung disease has multiple causes, usually classified by underlying risk factors. If no triggering factor can be elucidated, the diagnosis of idiopathic pulmonary fibrosis is often assigned.

TABLE A30. Major Categories of Interstitial Lung Disease (ILD)
Primary lung diseases Idiopathic pulmonary fibrosis* Sarcoidosis* Bronchiolitis obliterans with organizing pneumonia* Lymphocytic interstitial pneumonia Histiocytosis X Lymphangioleiomyomatosis
ILD associated with drugs or treatments Antibiotics* Anti-inflammatory agents Cardiovascular drugs* Antineoplastic agents* Illicit drugs Dietary supplements Oxygen Radiation Paraquat

Environment/occupation-associated ILD
Organic dusts/hypersensitivity pneumonitis
  (>40 known agents)
    Farmer's lung*
    Air conditioner-humidifier lung*
    Bird breeder's lung*
    Bagassosis
    Inorganic dusts
    Silicosis*
    Asbestosis*
    Coal workers' pneumoconiosis*
    Berylliosis
  Gases/fumes/vapors
    Oxides of nitrogen
    Sulfur dioxide
    Toluene diisocyanate
    Oxides of metals
    Hydrocarbons
    Thermosetting resins

ILD associated with systemic rheumatic disorder Rheumatoid arthritis* Systemic lupus erythematosus* Scleroderma* Polymyositis-dermatomyositis* Sjögren syndrome Mixed connective tissue disease* Ankylosing spondylitis
Alveolar filling disorders Diffuse alveolar hemorrhage Goodpasture syndrome Idiopathic pulmonary hemosiderosis Pulmonary alveolar proteinosis Chronic eosinophilic pneumonia*

TABLE A30. (Continued)
ILD associated with pulmonary vasculitis Wegener's granulomatosis Churg-Strauss syndrome Hypersensitivity vasculitis Necrotizing sarcoid granulomatosis
Inherited disorders Familial idiopathic pulmonary fibrosis Neurofibromatosis Tuberous sclerosis Gaucher disease Niemann-Pick disease Hermansky-Pudlak syndrome

*Disorders that are the most common causes of ILD or less common conditions in which ILD is a prominent manifestation of disease.

31–C, 32–E

Amiodarone, a cardiac antiarrhythmic drug used predominantly for treating ventricular dysrhythmias, causes interstitial lung disease in 5% to 10% of patients. Risk factors include maintenance doses of greater than 400 mg/day, previous pulmonary disease, concurrent cardiopulmonary bypass, oxygen therapy, or general anesthesia. The time it takes to develop amiodarone pneumonitis is variable, ranging from a few days to over a decade, but it is generally a few months to years. In practice, the disease can develop at any time during treatment with the drug. In rare instances, amiodarone pneumonitis may develop a few weeks or months after cessation, due to the long half-life of the drug in lung tissues. Amiodarone pneumonitis can result in different pulmonary syndromes, including subacute interstitial pneumonitis, migratory opacities of BOOP, ARDS, and multiple shaggy lung nodules. The diagnosis of amiodarone lung is favored if there are diffuse, often asymmetrical, interstitial opacities with a ground-glass pattern at high-resolution CT. Careful exclusion of left heart failure with pulmonary edema is required and the pulmonary function pattern is restrictive in nature, with reduced carbon monoxide transfer and hypoxemia, often severe and disproportionate to the extent of pulmonary opacities. Histology from a lung biopsy is the mainstay of diagnosis, as changes associated with amiodarone toxicity are distinctive; given the risks of this procedure, diagnosis is most often made clinically. The mainstay of therapy is withdrawal of the drug and prolonged steroid treatment, but the pulmonary fibrosis is usually irreversible.

33–E, 34–D, 35–D, 36–E

Because most endovascular infections in injection drug users are caused by *Staphylococcus aureus*, empiric therapy should include an antistaphylococcal penicillin (oxacillin or nafcillin) or vancomycin. The incidence of community-acquired methicillin-resistant *Staphylococcus aureus* (MRSA) infection is increasing, particularly in injection drug users; therefore, some experts favor using vancomycin, instead of an antistaphylococcal penicillin, until the results of blood culture and sensitivity are known. For right-sided (usually tricuspid valve) *S. aureus* native-valve endocarditis in an injection drug user, traditional therapy consists of 4 to 6 weeks of an antistaphylococcal penicillin, plus low-dose aminoglycoside (gentamicin or tobramycin at 1 mg/kg q8h) for the first 3 to 5 days of treatment. In patients with MRSA or a β-lactam allergy, vancomycin should be substituted for the penicillin. A useful alternative for injection drug users with methicillin-sensitive *Staphylococcus aureus* (MSSA) tricuspid valve endocarditis consists of 2 weeks of an antistaphylococcal penicillin with low-dose aminoglycoside for the entire duration of therapy. Patients with HIV infection or extrapulmonary embolic events should not receive short-course therapy. Vancomycin should not be used in 2-week regimens.

A set of clinical criteria, commonly known as the Duke criteria (Durack DT, Lukes AS, Bright DK, et al. Am J Med 1994;96:200) uses historic, physical, microbiologic, and echocardiographic data to accept or reject the diagnosis of infective endocarditis. A definitive diagnosis requires the presence of two major, or one major and three minor, or five minor criteria and carries an accuracy of 80%. Major criteria include the recovery of at least two separate blood cultures positive for a pathogen that typically causes endocarditis; the demonstration of a vegetation, myocardial abscess, or prosthetic valve dehiscence by echocardiogram; or a new regurgitant murmur by exam. Minor criteria include the presence of a condition that predisposes to infective endocarditis (such as injection drug use); temperature >38°C; embolic disease; immunologic phenomena such as Roth spots, glomerulonephritis, Osler nodes, or rheumatoid factor; positive blood cultures not meeting the requirements of a major criterion; or an echocardiographic finding not meeting the requirements of a major criterion. The diagnosis of infective endocarditis can be rejected if these criteria are not met, if an alternative source of infection is found, or if the patient has defervesced with 4 or 5 days of antibiotics.

Patient I.E. has one major (positive blood cultures with a likely pathogen) and three minor (a predisposing condition, fever >38°C, and pulmonary emboli) criteria. It is highly likely that she has infective endocarditis, and that the tricuspid valve is the site of her infection. (Pulmonary emboli arise from right-sided disease, or left-sided disease with a patent foramen ovale; the tricuspid valve is more often infected than the pulmonic valve.) Many clinicians would stop the workup at this point and treat accordingly. Others would confirm the diagnosis with a TEE. Because of its low sensitivity, a transthoracic echocardiogram (TTE) should not be used to rule out endocarditis.

S. aureus septic thrombophlebitis of a deep vein could also explain all of patient's I.E.'s presenting symptoms, including her pulmonary emboli. Treatment includes 4 to 6 weeks of antibiotics and, usually, anticoagulation. A vascular surgeon should be consulted to evaluate the possibility of thrombectomy.

Finally, hospitalization can provide the opportunity to offer an injection drug user preventive medical care, as well as entry into a substance abuse rehabilitation program. Methadone will help control this patient's withdrawal symptoms, but an acute hospitalization is not the best place to begin methadone therapy to help wean her off heroin. Rather, discharge to a rehabilitation facility where it can be begun is in order. Buprenorphine, a mixed opioid agonist/antagonist, is useful in treating heroin withdrawal while the patient is hospitalized.

37–E, 38–C, 39–A, 40–D

In addition to chest x-ray, CBC with differential, serum chemistries, oxygen saturation, and ABG, the Infectious Diseases Society of America (IDSA) recommendations for the evaluation of CAP in hospitalized adults include collecting two sets of blood cultures as well as a high-quality expectorated sputum for Gram stain and culture before starting antibiotics. Some respected authorities discount the use of sputum microbiology in managing CAP because it can often be contaminated by oral flora and has never (in retrospective studies only) been shown to decrease mortality. Nevertheless, the IDSA holds that a high-quality sputum sample, processed quickly and interpreted by experienced personnel, is sufficiently sensitive and specific to guide antibiotic use and track antimicrobial resistance, benefiting the health of both the patient and the public.

A high-quality sputum sample should be obtained by deep cough in the presence of a health care provider and should appear purulent. It should contain <10 squamous epithelial cells and >25 PMNs per low-power field. It should be rapidly transported to the lab (preferably in the hands of the person who obtained the sample). Blood cultures can be a useful adjunct to sputum studies, as they are positive for the pathogen responsible for pneumonia in 10% of patients. Finally, sending HIV serology should be considered in all patients who are 15 to 54 years old with CAP. Testing for TB, legionella, and/or bronchoscopy should be considered for any patient with CAP who does not respond to appropriate empiric antibiotic therapy.

Most bacterial CAP is caused by *Streptococcus pneumoniae, Haemophilus influenzae,* and the so-called atypical pathogens (e.g., *Mycoplasma pneumoniae, Chlamydia pneumoniae, Moraxella catarrhalis*), and less often *Klebsiella pneumoniae* or *Staphylococcus aureus.* The appropriate empiric therapy of patients ill enough to be hospitalized should cover the pneumococcus, atypicals, and community-acquired gram-negative rods (GNRs). Ceftriaxone or cefotaxime, and β-lactam/β-lactamase inhibitors are active against streptococci and GNRs; and the macrolides, tetracycline, and all fluoroquinolones cover atypicals. Levofloxacin and moxifloxacin are two fluoroquinolones active against streptococci, GNRs, and atypicals. There is evidence, however, of ciprofloxacin failing against the pneumococcus. The emergence of both intermediate and high-level penicillin resistance in the pneumococcus is a serious worldwide problem. Cefotaxime, ceftriaxone, and the antistreptococcal fluoroquinolones remain reliably active against intermediate-level penicillin-resistant pneumococci (MIC of penicillin, 0.1–1.0 μg/mL), but any patient with high-level penicillin resistance should receive vancomycin.

The standard recommended duration of antibiotic therapy for pneumococcal CAP is until 3 to 5 days after the patient has defervesced.

Pneumocystis carinii pneumonia (PCP), common in patients with AIDS and fewer than 200 CD4+ T cells, is the most common AIDS-defining illness, and may therefore masquerade as CAP in patients unaware of their HIV infection. In addition to having a more prolonged onset than CAP, classic PCP presentation includes bilateral interstitial infiltrates with a ground-glass appearance on chest x-ray. Nevertheless, PCP can resemble almost any type of infiltrate radiologically, although it is not known to present with pleural effusions. In fact, up to 30% of patients with PCP may present with radiologically clear lung fields.

41–F, 42–C, 43–A, 44–C

The acute management of patients with atrial fibrillation depends on several pieces of information: the patient's hemodynamic stability; the estimated duration of the arrhythmia; and the presence of certain precipitating causes that would require immediate attention. The two most dangerous threats posed by atrial fibrillation acutely are embolization from a left atrial thrombus, and hemodynamic instability due to an unsustainable rapid ventricular response. The probability of an atrial thrombus forming increases after 24 to 48 hours of atrial fibrillation. The danger of immediate cardioversion is that the change from fibrillation to sinus rhythm could dislodge atrial thrombus. Therefore, in a hemodynamically stable patient whose atrial fibrillation is of uncertain duration (such as the patient described here), an initial approach would be to control the ventricular heart rate with diltiazem or a beta-blocker such as metoprolol or esmolol, and start anticoagulation. Digoxin can also be used to slow ventricular response, but is less effective, particularly with patient activity. Congestive heart failure can occur as a result of atrial fibrillation, due either to cardiomyopathy from sustained rapid response, or to the decrease in cardiac output from the loss of adequate ventricular filling from the atrium. Congestive heart failure can also precipitate atrial fibrillation. In either event, symptomatic relief can be provided with diuresis. Most patients with atrial fibrillation who require anticoagulation are treated with warfarin. Patients with paroxysmal atrial fibrillation in the absence of underlying cardiac disease, who are younger than 65 years old, and do not have risk factors for stroke that are associated with atrial fibrillation (mitral stenosis, hypertension, previous TIA or CVA, CHF, left ventricular dysfunction), are sometimes prophylactically anticoagulated with aspirin rather than warfarin.

It is important to identify and treat causes of secondary atrial fibrillation. Therefore in this patient, TSH, cardiac enzymes, an echocardiogram, and investigation of the patient's alcohol consumption would be helpful.

It is not always possible to restore and maintain sinus rhythm in a patient with atrial fibrillation. Some asymptomatic patients are managed

ANSWERS

long term with rate-controlling drugs and anti-coagulation. Nevertheless, it is a generally accepted strategy to try to restore sinus rhythm in patients with new onset atrial fibrillation. There are two strategies for cardioversion of patients with recent onset atrial fibrillation of unknown duration. The traditional approach consists of anticoagulation for 3 weeks, followed by pharmacologic or direct-current cardioversion with or without antiarrhythmic medication, followed by an additional 6 to 12 weeks of anticoagulation. A recent alternative approach has been to start anticoagulation, rule out atrial thrombus with a transesophageal echocardiogram, and then cardiovert immediately, followed by 6 to 12 weeks of additional anticoagulation (Manning WJ, Silverman DI, Keighley CS, et al. J Am Coll Cardiol 1995;25:1354–61). Should either approach fail to maintain sinus rhythm, cardioversion can be repeated. Strategies for the treatment of recurrent, sustained atrial fibrillation include long-term anticoagulation plus pharmacologic rate control or antiarrhythmic therapy, or ablation of the AV node and placement of a pacemaker.

45–E

ST segment *elevations* almost always indicate ongoing myocardial damage due to total occlusion of a coronary artery, known as a "Q wave" MI (myocarditis can also cause ST elevation, but this is usually across all leads, and with a characteristic shape). Evidence of an ongoing Q wave infarction requires an immediate attempt at reperfusion with thrombolytics, angioplasty, or in some cases emergent bypass surgery. ST segment *depressions* or *T wave inversions* indicate myocardial ischemia, generally due to subtotal occlusion of a coronary artery. Such an event may end in some degree of myocardial damage (non-Q wave MI) if there is an elevation in serum myocardial enzymes, or in spontaneous reperfusion (unstable angina) if there is no enzyme elevation. From the ECG, this patient could be experiencing either unstable angina or a non-Q wave MI.

46–D

The number of drugs and procedures now used to treat the acute coronary syndromes (and the number and names of the trials demonstrating their effectiveness) can seem overwhelming. If you remember, however, that the aggregation of activated platelets at the site of a ruptured coronary plaque occludes the artery, which decreases

blood flow to downstream myocardium, which produces ischemia and subsequent muscle damage, then the treatments make sense. *Aspirin* and *heparin* inhibit platelet activation and thrombus formation; supplemental *oxygen* may benefit ischemic myocardium; *nitrates* decrease myocardial oxygen demand by lowering preload and dilating coronary vessels; and *beta-blockers* decrease myocardial workload by lowering heart rate, and may protect against ischemia-induced arrhythmias as well. Continuous monitoring of vital signs and the ECG assesses the effectiveness of treatment and warns of evolving disease. Serial measurement of cardiac troponins and creatine kinase (CK-MB) distinguishes non-Q wave MI from unstable angina. Monitoring the aPTT and platelet count is necessary for adjusting the dose of unfractionated heparin and checking for heparin-induced thrombocytopenia (HIT). Because thrombolytic agents *increase* patient mortality in unstable angina and non-Q wave MI, they are currently contraindicated in these acute coronary syndromes, but remain vitally important in the treatment of Q wave MI.

47–D

Patients with unstable angina who remain symptomatic after 30 minutes of conventional therapy are at increased risk of MI, pulmonary edema, arrhythmias, and death. In addition to maximal tolerated medical therapy and intensive hemodynamic monitoring, they should be considered for emergent cardiac catheterization and percutaneous transluminal coronary angioplasty (PTCA). The administration of glycoprotein IIb/IIIa inhibitors, which block platelet aggregation, has improved the outcome of coronary occlusions treated with PTCA and stenting. These agents are also under study for use without PTCA in the initial management of unstable angina.

48–C

Patients with unstable angina who respond to initial treatment, and are hemodynamically stable and free of ischemic signs and symptoms for 24 hours, can be transferred to less intensive medical treatment. This includes discontinuing continuous cardiac monitoring, and converting IV medications to oral. Serial measurement of cardiac enzymes should continue until an MI has been ruled out. Heparin is usually continued for 2 days after cessation of pain. Subsequent management can either be invasive or conservative, as described in the question.

49–B

Surgical repair is indicated for severe acute aortic dissection, especially in the setting of probable vascular compromise, as indicated by reduced femoral pulses and evidence of hypoperfusion to the spinal arteries with paraparesis and paresthesias in the lower extremities. The rise in creatinine may be secondary to compromise of one or both renal arteries. Thus, halting the progression of the dissecting hematoma will prevent lethal complications. Indeed, aortic dissection has a high mortality: more than 25% of all patients die within the first 24 hours after the onset of dissection, more than 50% die within the first week, more than 75% die within 1 month, and more than 90% die within 1 year without treatment. "Chronic" aortic dissections (present for more than 2 weeks) may not need immediate surgical repair and can even be solely medically managed depending on the clinical situation. Severe acute aortic dissection may need to be temporarily medically managed while surgical repair is being arranged: management of pain and the reduction of systolic blood pressure to 100–120 mmHg with short-acting agents is essential. Hypertensive control is usually achieved with a combination of a sodium nitroprusside drip and a short-acting beta blocker.

50–D

The diagnosis of aortic dissection is usually made with one of four imaging modalities: aortography, contrast-enhanced CT, MRI, and echocardiography. Aortography was formerly the gold standard, but it has fallen out of favor because of the risks of the procedure, the duration, and the need to transport an unstable patient to the angiography suite. Spiral (helical) contrast-enhanced CT is non-invasive and quick, though it rarely identifies the actual site of the intimal tear. MRI is noninvasive and does not require contrast, but metal cannot be placed in the MRI scanner and the procedure involves transport of unstable patients. Trans-thoracic echocardiography has a poor sensitivity but transesophageal echocardiography allows efficiency and bedside diagnosis. The method of imaging used often depends on the stability of the patient, the resources of the hospital, and the clinical targeting of the dissection location.

51–E

Any disease process that undermines the integrity of the elastic or muscular components of the media predisposes the aorta to dissection. Cystic medial degeneration is an intrinsic feature of several hereditary defects of connective tissue, most notably the Marfan and Ehlers-Danlos syndromes. Indeed, Marfan syndrome accounts for 5% to 9% of all aortic dissections. Hypertension and atherosclerotic disease also predispose patients to aortic dissection. A bicuspid aortic valve is a well-established risk factor for proximal aortic dissection and has historically been found in 7% to 14% of all aortic dissections, but the risk of the latter is independent of the severity of the bicuspid valve stenosis. Coarctation of the aorta, arteritis, and aortic involvement by tertiary syphilis also predispose the aorta to dissection. An unexplained relationship between pregnancy and aortic dissection exists, and direct trauma to the aorta may also cause dissection. The Eaton-Lambert syndrome is a disorder of the neuromuscular junction and does not predispose an individual to aortic dissection.

52–C

Aortic regurgitation is a frequent complication of proximal aortic dissection, with the murmur detected in 32% of cases. The dissection may dilate the aortic root so that the leaflets of the aortic valve are unable to coapt properly in diastole; the dissection may detach one or more aortic leaflets from their commissural attachments; or the intimal flap may prolapse into the LV outflow tract, preventing aortic valve closure.

53–D, 54–B

The only effective therapy for severe aortic stenosis is aortic valve replacement (AVR). Valve replacement can return survival completely to normal from the dire predictions without treatment, even in the presence of symptoms. Even octogenarians benefit from AVR; unless other comorbid factors preclude surgery, age should not be a contraindication to valve replacement. Reduced ejection fraction should also not be a contraindication for AVR, as the ejection fraction can dramatically improve after surgery when the excess afterload imposed by the stenotic valve is relieved. In acquired aortic stenosis, the valves are usually heavily calcific, and balloon valvuloplasty is relatively ineffective. Indeed, survival following this procedure is similar to that of untreated patients. Balloon valvuloplasty is thus used only palliatively or as a bridging measure to surgery. There is no effective medical therapy for severe aortic stenosis. Vasodilators, such as calcium channel blockers and ACE inhibitors, may

ANSWERS

serve to reduce afterload and increase flow through the stenotic valve, but may also reduce preload, leading to decreased flow to the diseased valve, decreased cardiac output, and syncope. Beta-blockers can depress myocardial function and induce LV failure and should be avoided in patients with aortic stenosis. Diuretics can be used cautiously in patients with heart failure while awaiting valve replacement, and digitalis may improve myocardial function. Antibiotic prophylactic therapy for bacterial endocarditis is indicated in aortic stenosis.

55–B

Approximately 1% of the population is born with a bicuspid aortic valve, with a male predominance to this condition. These valves tend to deteriorate with age, with one-third of such valves becoming stenotic, one-third becoming regurgitant, and the remainder causing only minor hemodynamic abnormalities. In terms of the development of aortic stenosis, the architecture of the bicuspid flow induces turbulent flow, leading to fibrosis, calcification of the leaflets, and narrowing of the aortic orifice into adulthood. The development of aortic stenosis in the presence of a bicuspid valve usually occurs in the fourth, fifth, and sixth decades of life, as compared to the development of aortic stenosis in normal tricuspid valves in the sixth to eighth decades of life. The congenital defect of a unicuspid valve usually produces severe obstruction in infancy.

56–C

The pulse in aortic stenosis has a slow rise with less volume, known as pulsus parvus et tardus.

57–D

The approach to a patient with suspected acute myocardial infarction (MI) depends on the type of infarct—left ventricular, right ventricular, Q wave, or non-Q wave. The patient in this case is experiencing an acute left ventricular Q wave MI. Most cases of acute left ventricular Q wave infarction can be presumptively diagnosed by the electrocardiographic finding of ST segment elevation >1 mm in two or more contiguous leads, or by new left bundle branch block (LBBB), and *usually but not always* by substernal chest pain. Elevated cardiac enzymes (CK-MB and troponins) subsequently confirm the diagnosis. The pathophysiology of Q wave infarction involves

occlusion of the epicardial coronary arteries supplying the myocardium; the amount of myocardial damage, and the subsequent cardiac morbidity and mortality depend greatly on the duration of ischemia. Therefore, ECG evidence of acute Q wave LV infarct should prompt an attempt at coronary reperfusion as soon as possible, as well as medical therapy to limit infarct size and relieve pain. Medical thrombolysis is indicated for all patients with ST elevation or new LBBB who present within 12 hours of the onset of symptoms, without cardiogenic shock or contraindications to thrombolytics. Primary PTCA is indicated under the same conditions, as long as it can be performed within 90 minutes of presentation to the hospital by experienced operators with surgical backup, and in patients whose pain has lasted more than 12 hours, or who present in cardiogenic shock or with contraindications to thrombolysis.

58–D

Successful reperfusion is accompanied by rapid resolution of pain, conversion of ST elevation to Q waves, and often the transient occurrence of non-life-threatening idioventricular arrhythmias. Unless contraindicated by hypotension or bradycardia, ACE inhibitors and beta-blockers should be started within the first 24 hours of hospitalization to limit infarct size and incidence of arrhythmia, and ACE-inhibitors should be continued indefinitely for patients with significant LV dysfunction. If tPA was chosen for thrombolysis, heparin should be continued for 24 to 48 hours. Further diagnostic testing of patients with acute MI treated with thrombolysis, also known as risk-stratification for further ischemic events, is the subject of much discussion. The ACC/AHA guidelines recommend classifying patients by their risk of ischemic events at discharge. Those at high risk include patients with ongoing symptomatic or electrocardiographic ischemia; LV ejection fraction <40%; sustained ventricular arrhythmias; history of prior MI; age >70 years; diabetes; and evidence of pulmonary edema on examination or chest radiogram. Patients at high risk should undergo predischarge angiography to determine their suitability for revascularization. Those at lower risk of cardiac events can undergo symptom-limited exercise treadmill testing (ETT) 2 to 3 weeks after discharge, or submaximal ETT shortly before discharge. The results of either type of ETT then determine whether the patient will receive cardiac catheterization, noninvasive imaging studies, or continued medical therapy. Electrophysiologic testing is reserved for patients who are at higher risk of sudden cardiac death after discharge (i.e., those who experience ventricular fibrillation after the first 48 hours of hospitalization). Assuming that they are free of CHF, conduction disease, or ventricular aneurysm, patients who experience transient ventricular fibrillation early in ischemia (i.e., within 24 hours) are at increased risk of in-hospital death but not thereafter, and do not require electrophysiologic testing.

59–C

This patient's symptoms indicate recurrent ischemia, which can either consist of postinfarction angina or recurrent MI. The ECG confirms the latter. Thirty percent of patients who undergo initially successful thrombolysis experience postinfarction angina, and 10% experience early reinfarction. Although repeat thrombolysis is an option, such postinfarction ischemia usually indicates the need for catheterization, to define the patient's coronary anatomy, followed by revascularization. All such patients should receive maximal medical therapy as well.

60–E

The secondary prevention of MI decreases the risk of death and reinfarction. It consists of aspirin, at least 2 years of beta-blockade, indefinite ACE inhibitor therapy in those with significantly lowered ejection fraction or large regional wall-motion abnormality, and risk factor modification. The latter includes smoking cessation, control of hypertension, and reduction of LDL cholesterol to below 100 mg/dL.

61–E

Before you have performed any diagnostic test, even a resting 12-lead ECG, you must consider the relatively high probability that chest pain in a middle-aged man with hypertension represents coronary ischemia—the consequences of missing an ischemic event are grave. For this reason, and because a small percentage of ischemic events are electrocardiographically silent, it is important to keep an acute coronary syndrome at the top of the list of possible diagnoses, even though there are no ischemic ECG changes during the patient's chest pain.

Like angina, the pain of esophageal spasm is often described as crushing, with radiation to the upper extremities, and is relieved by nitroglycerin.

Esophageal spasm is neither common nor life-threatening, so it is important to evaluate more serious alternatives. Aortic dissection can present with sudden, intense, ripping chest pain radiating to the back; often both pulse and blood pressure differ considerably between the right and left arms, and the pain is difficult to control. The patient's history, examination, and response to therapy make aortic dissection unlikely. Pulmonary embolism is notoriously difficult to diagnose, and can present nonspecifically as chest pain with tachycardia. It should not respond to nitroglycerin, however.

62–D, 63–B, 64–C

The possible causes of chest pain in this patient are too serious to allow him to go home before further evaluation (unless he refuses to stay). At the same time, his pain is not so clearly cardiac as to warrant immediate cardiac catheterization. Of the choices listed, a reasonable approach would be to monitor him in the hospital with serial sampling of his cardiac enzymes (CK-MB and troponin) and serial ECGs to make sure he is not experiencing an acute coronary syndrome, and to perform noninvasive diagnostic testing such as a stress ECG once the diagnosis of acute MI has been ruled out. To accomplish this, the patient can either be admitted to the hospital overnight or be observed in a specialized chest-pain unit (the latter is increasingly a part of many EDs due to the high prevalence of nonspecific chest pain). Because cardiac troponins remain elevated for 7 to 14 days after myocardial damage, a single measurement does not help diagnose an acute event. Although the results of a fasting lipid profile would not change the acute management of this patient, they might provide the basis for preventive lipid-lowering therapy after discharge. A chest x-ray is easy to obtain and would rule out some thoracic causes of chest pain such as pleural masses, a small pneumothorax, or pneumonia. Once you are satisfied that the patient's chest pain is not caused by ischemia or other serious conditions, a barium swallow would help begin the workup for esophageal spasm.

65–E

Contributing factors to GERD include caffeinated products, peppermint, tobacco, ethanol, chocolate, and foods with high concentrations of fat or carbohydrate, all of which decrease LES pressure and increase heartburn. Citrus fruits, other fruit juices, and tomato-based products often exacerbate symptoms. Although pregnancy may cause reflux because of increased intra-abdominal pressure, the primary reason for heartburn in pregnancy is reduced sphincter pressure as a consequence of increased circulating levels of progesterone and estrogen. Reflux can be precipitated in normal persons by exercise, with jogging after meals as the most common cause.

66–C

A strong, dose-related, independent risk for adenocarcinoma of the esophagus is conferred by symptomatic gastroesophageal reflux. In a substantial number of patients with long-standing severe reflux, a premalignant change develops that is referred to as Barrett's esophagus, which denotes metaplastic columnar epithelialization of the distal esophagus. Barrett's esophagus is believed to represent a reparative response to tissue injury from chronic exposure to gastric acid, pepsin, and bile (annual incidence, 0.6% per year; prevalence, 10% among those with reflux lasting longer than 20 years). Histologically, the normal stratified squamous epithelium of the mucosa is replaced by columnar epithelium. Dysplastic transformation may ensue and eventually lead to adenocarcinoma. The risk for the development of adenocarcinoma with onset of Barrett's esophagus is less than 1% annually but rises fivefold with the onset of low-grade dysplasia and 10-fold in persons with high-grade dysplasia. Symptoms of both Barrett's esophagus and adenocarcinoma are the same as those of GERD, which was the reasoning for endoscopic screening of this patient.

Other complications of GERD include severe erosive esophagitis or stricture formation, resulting in dysphagia or odynophagia. Esophageal hemorrhage can occur, resulting in either a slow chronic bleeding process or a brisk hematemesis. Reflux-induced asthma and laryngitis are among the airway consequences of chronic GERD. Unexplained wheezing, voice change, chronic cough, and a lump in the throat are among the symptoms reported; reflux must be considered when such complaints develop in the absence of a known cause. Dental erosions occur in a substantial proportion of patients with marked reflux as a consequence of the effects of acid and bile on tooth enamel.

67–E, 68–D

Clinicians now advocate a five-stage management strategy for GERD, with the various modalities outlined in Table A67. In terms of pharmacologic therapy, patients should first be tried on antacids and H_2-receptor antagonists. However, clinical trials have shown that proton pump inhibitors provide better symptom control, esophageal healing, and maintenance of remission in GERD than the other known agents. Omeprazole and lansoprazole are the currently available proton pump inhibitors. These drugs strongly inhibit gastric acid secretion by irreversibly inhibiting the H^+-K^+ adenosine triphosphatase pump of the parietal cell. By blocking the final common pathway of gastric acid secretion, the proton pump inhibitors provide a greater degree and duration of gastric acid suppression compared with H_2-receptor blockade. Long-term use of proton pump inhibitors in humans has not been associated with an increased risk of gastric carcinoma, although this was initially a concern from animal studies. Prolonged use of the drugs has been associated with gastric atrophy; however, atrophy is more likely to be a problem in patients infected with *Helicobacter pylori*. The proton pump inhibitors are fairly well tolerated, with the most common side effects being nausea, diarrhea, constipation, headache, and skin rash. Omeprazole and lansoprazole are more expensive than standard-dose H_2-receptor blockers or prokinetic agents. However, when prescribed appropriately to patients with severe symptoms or refractory disease, they are more cost-effective because of their higher healing and remission rates and the consequent prevention of complications.

TABLE A67. Management Stages for Gastroesophageal Reflux Disease

Stage I: Lifestyle modification (elevate head of bed; reduce weight; modify diet to decrease consumption of fatty foods, spicy foods, and caffeine; smoking cessation; avoid recumbency post-prandially)

Stage II: Over-the-counter medication as needed (magnesium or aluminum-containing antacids; H_2-receptor blockade)

Stage III: Scheduled medication treatment (H_2-blockers or prokinetic agents for 8 to 12 weeks; if symptoms persist, high-dose H_2-blockers or proton pump inhibitors for another 8 to 12 weeks; can use proton pump inhibitors as first-line agent if erosive esophagitis is present)

Stage IV: Maintenance therapy (for patients with persistent or complicated disease, continue lowest dose possible of H_2-blocker or proton pump inhibitor)

Stage V: Surgery (may be indicated for patients with erosive esophagitis, severe symptoms or disease complications: laparoscopic Nissen or Toupet fundoplication procedure)

69–B, 70–D, 71–B

In the initial approach to a GI bleed, stabilizing the patient and evaluating the cause of the bleed are simultaneous, with the former assuming greater importance. The patient's hemodynamic state should be assessed with orthostatic blood pressure and heart rate measurements, and an estimate of jugular venous pressure (JVP). The potential need for rapid, large volume resuscitation with IV fluids and blood should be addressed by placing at least two large-bore peripheral IV lines, typing and crossmatching the patient's blood for transfusion, and checking a coagulation profile and serial hematocrits. Although central lines often have several lumens, their length and narrow gauge slow the infusion of fluids. Because short, fat peripheral lines offer far less resistance, they are useful in resuscitations. Additionally, because it can take at least 8 hours for the hematocrit to re-equilibrate after a bleed, the initial hematocrit usually underestimates the percentage of blood volume lost; so serial measurements are important. In general, a goal for transfusion therapy is to maintain a hematocrit of 25% to 30%.

If there is a possibility that the bleed is coming from the upper GI tract, then gastric lavage with room-temperature saline through an NG or OG tube can be very useful in assessing the activity of the bleed (and the urgency of treatment), and preparing the upper GI tract for endoscopy. A finding of clear or bilious fluid in an NG aspirate means that an active bleed is unlikely. The finding of coffee-ground material or blood signals an active bleed, and requires urgent EGD to find the source and, in many cases, stop the bleeding. The usual practice is to continue lavage and aspiration until the aspirate runs clear, while recording the amount of saline required to reach this point. Failure of the blood to clear signifies persistent bleed and requires EGD as soon as possible. The most common causes of upper GI bleed are duodenal and gastric ulcer disease, erosive gastropathy, bleeding esophageal varices associated with portal hypertension, gastroesophageal junction (Mallory-Weiss) tears, and vascular malformations. Treatment varies by cause; many lesions can be sclerosed, banded, or injected with epinephrine during EGD. Gastropathy often responds to pharmacologic H_2 or proton pump inhibition.

72–B

Hemodynamic stabilization and resuscitation are also important first steps in the approach to a suspected lower GI bleed. The possibility of an upper GI bleed should still be evaluated by NG lavage; often the workup for a lower GI bleed includes EGD to rule out an upper source.

Anoscopy can be employed to look for bleeding hemorrhoids or fissures. A stable, intermittently bleeding patient can be evaluated with elective colonoscopy after lower GI tract lavage with an electrolyte solution. An actively bleeding patient stable enough to tolerate it can get lavage followed by urgent colonoscopy, and/or radiolabeled RBC scan or mesenteric angiogram to localize the source of the bleed. Once the source is found, it can be treated by colonoscopic cautery, angiographic embolization, or surgery. It should be obvious from this general outline that early involvement of gastroenterologists and surgeons is essential; these specialists are much more helpful if you have already stabilized the patient and evaluated the possible sources of the bleed.

73–C, 74–B

The ultrasound confirms that this patient has acute cholecystitis. A regimen of intravenous rehydration, analgesia, and antibiotics will usually relieve an acute episode of cholecystitis. Although not every episode of cystic duct obstruction involves bacterial superinfection, therapy that covers Enterobacteriaceae and anaerobes ± enterococci is recommended. Commonly used regimens include monotherapy with a β-lactam/β-lactamase inhibitor; dual therapy with a third-generation cephalosporin plus metronidazole; or triple therapy with ampicillin, metronidazole, and either an aminoglycoside or a fluoroquinolone. It is important to remember that cephalosporins do not treat enterococcal infections. Because of the high risk of recurrent cholecystitis, early cholecystectomy (within 2 to 3 days after hospitalization) should be performed. Low morbidity and mortality make laparoscopic cholecystectomy the procedure of choice; should complications arise during surgery, the operation can be converted to an open procedure. Patients who are unable to undergo cholecystectomy can be treated with percutaneous cholecystostomy. Emergent cholecystectomy, which carries a higher risk of mortality, is nevertheless indicated for patients with patients with perforation or gangrene of the gallbladder.

75–C, 76–A

The patient now presents with fevers and chills, jaundice, and RUQ pain, otherwise known as Charcot's triad. This is the classic presentation of cholangitis due to obstruction of the common bile duct. Such an obstruction is often caused by a stone (choledocholithiasis), and can occur in

ANSWERS

patients with or without a gallbladder. Common bile duct obstruction can also arise from a tumor of the common duct, or from extrinsic compression, such as metastatic or regional malignancy. Cholangitis accompanied by signs of sepsis or altered mental status suggests pus in the biliary tree, which has a high mortality and requires emergent drainage. Choledocholithiasis is associated with higher bilirubin, transaminases, and alkaline phosphatase levels than cholecystitis. The approach to a patient suspected of having cholangitis includes blood cultures, antibiotics that cover gram-positive, gram-negative, and anaerobic bacteria, and urgent drainage. ERCP provides both definitive diagnosis and treatment via papillotomy and stone removal.

77–E

The curved (comma or S-shaped) gram-negative organisms are most likely *Campylobacter jejuni*, given their typical morphology. *Campylobacter* causes an inflammatory diarrhea thought to be secondary to enterotoxin production along with mucosal invasion. Systemic symptoms such as fever, nausea, and malaise are often present along with the typical bacterial diarrheal symptoms of severe abdominal pain and bloody stool with mucus. Although ciprofloxacin is usually the initial treatment for *Campylobacter* infections, there are increasing rates of fluoroquinolone-resistance from areas around the world, most prominently Southeast Asia and Spain due to use of quinolones in animal feed. The treatment of choice for ciprofloxacin-resistant *Campylobacter* is a macrolide, such as azithromycin.

78–C

Recommendations for avoiding traveler's diarrhea include drinking only boiled, bottled, or treated water; avoiding ice; and avoiding salads, raw vegetables, and unpeeled fruits; as well as trying to eat hot, freshly cooked foods. Prophylactic antimicrobial agents are not generally recommended, given the side effects from antibiotic therapy and the danger of developing drug-resistant bacteria. However, some clinicians advocate prophylactic use of bismuth subsalicylate, which has some antibacterial properties, in the setting of travel.

79–B, 80–D

The organism most typically associated with drinking from freshwater streams is *Giardia lamblia,* a parasite that usually causes inflammation of the duodenal mucosa, leading to malabsorption of protein and fat. Symptoms thus include non-bloody, foul-smelling, large-volume diarrhea, accompanied by nausea, anorexia, flatulence, and abdominal cramps that can persist for weeks or months. Diagnosis is made by finding trophozoites or cysts of the organism in stools (Figure A80). The treatment of choice is metronidazole orally. Prevention involves drinking boiled, filtered, or iodine-treated water in endemic areas and while hiking.

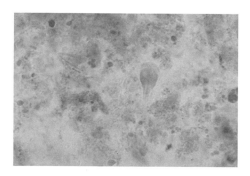

FIGURE A80 *Giardia lamblia* trophozoite stained by trichrome. (Image provided by Dr. Mae Melvin at the Centers for Disease Control; public domain: phil.cdc.gov.)

81–D, 82–E, 83–B, 84–E

In Crohn's disease (CD), inflammation extends through the full thickness of the bowel wall, often with granulomas, and can involve any section of the GI tract, with intervening areas of normal mucosa (hence the term skip lesions). In addition, because of the transmural nature of the disease, some patients with CD develop enteroenteric, enterovesicular, enterovaginal, or enterocutaneous fistulas, as well as intra-abdominal abscesses. Colonic granulomas are much more common in CD than in ulcerative colitis (UC). Hemorrhage and bloody diarrhea are less common in CD than in UC. Colonoscopy and upper GI tract radiography can reveal the bowel segments involved in Crohn disease, as well as the presence of fistulas.

Ulcerative colitis always involves the rectosigmoid area, with signs of edema, friable mucosa, and erosions. It may also extend proximally along the colon, but never involves the small bowel or shows skip lesions. Therefore, sigmoidoscopy/colonoscopy are key to diagnosis. Barium enema can precipitate toxic megacolon in severe cases of UC.

A recent serologic protocol has proven to be helpful when the combination of clinical and endoscopic/radiographic features cannot distinguish between Crohn disease and ulcerative colitis. The combination of a negative pANCA and a positive ASCA is 50% sensitive and 97% specific for Crohn's disease, while the combination of a positive pANCA and negative ASCA is 57% sensitive and 97% specific for ulcerative colitis (Quinton JF, Sendid B, Reumauz D, et al. Gut 1998;42:788–91).

Systemic (corticosteroid) and topical (5-ASA-derived) anti-inflammatory agents are used to treat both CD and UC. Because CD often causes transmural lesions, antibiotics are used more commonly in CD than in UC. Furthermore, because CD may recur anywhere along the GI tract, surgery is reserved for occasions when medical management has failed, whereas a prophylactic colectomy is not uncommon after a series of symptomatic flares in UC because it is curative. Antimetabolites are used in CD, whereas cyclosporine is used in UC. Finally, the use of anti-TNF antibodies has recently been shown to dramatically improve the course of Crohn's disease complicated by fistulas.

85–B, 86–C, 87–C

The patient now has an examination suggesting an acute abdomen. In addition, he is tachycardic and tachypneic, and his blood pressure has actually decreased after 1 liter of IV fluids. Peritonitis, perforated viscus, and bowel infarction with necrosis, all life-threatening and rapidly progressive, are of the greatest concern. Repeating the CBC and chemistries and determining the arterial blood gas will alert you to a rising WBC, abnormal acid–base status, and positive anion gap, all of which can be seen in abdominal catastrophe. A repeat KUB can check for intestinal distention and perforation (the latter if subdiaphragmatic free air is present). Although abdominal CT scanning can be very helpful in detecting intra-abdominal emergencies, it may take too long to arrange in this situation, and should not preclude more readily available diagnostic information and emergent consultation with a general surgeon.

The pH of 7.27 indicates an acidosis. Calculating the anion gap, and plugging the serum bicarbonate and $PaCO_2$ into Winter's formula, shows that this is an anion gap metabolic acidosis with respiratory compensation. The mnemonic MUDPILES (Methanol, Uremia, Diabetic and alcoholic ketoacidosis, Paraldehyde, Iron and INH, Lactate, Ethylene glycol, Salicylate) for the causes of this type of acid–base disorder remind you that the possibility of lactic acidosis seems quite high, when coupled with the patient's abdominal examination and leukocytosis. Lactic acidosis is

often seen in bowel necrosis, and is an ominous finding. It can be confirmed by sending a serum sample to the clinical lab, but you should not wait for the results of this test before calling the surgeons, because the suspicion of necrotic bowel is enough reason to perform an emergent exploratory laparotomy.

88–D

Determining the precise cause of an acute abdomen before surgery is not always possible. Nevertheless, of the choices presented, infarcted bowel due to acute mesenteric ischemia seems the most likely. The early clinical presentation, namely periumbilical pain out of proportion to examination with rapid progression to generalized pain, is classic for acute mesenteric ischemia. The normal KUB rules out toxic megacolon, and the lack of antibiotic exposure makes a diagnosis of C. difficile-associated pseudomembranous colitis extremely unlikely. Acute mesenteric ischemia is usually caused by embolic or vasculitic obstruction of the superior mesenteric artery (SMA) or vein (SMV). Patients with fixed atherosclerotic disease of the SMA can also develop acute mesenteric ischemia when subjected to states of systemic hypoperfusion, such as hemorrhage or sepsis. Mesenteric ischemia should be suspected in patients with abdominal pain, as early diagnosis by angiography or mesenteric ultrasound improves survival; this condition progresses rapidly to small bowel infarction and necrosis, which carries a high mortality rate. Ischemic colitis, heralded by lower abdominal cramping and bloody diarrhea, is less immediately dangerous than small bowel ischemia, given the presence of collateral circulation, and can be confirmed by colonoscopy.

89–D, 90–C

The most likely diagnosis in this particular case is candidal esophagitis, given the whitish plaques on the mucosal surface of the esophagus (which probably represent confluent yeast colonies) and the pseudohyphae seen on biopsy examination. Additional evidence includes the patient's abundant oral thrush. Candidal esophagitis is one of the most common etiologies of odynophagia in AIDS and can usually be treated with fluconazole (100–200 mg PO QD) if the patient can tolerate oral medications (IV fluconazole can be administered if pills are not tolerated). This condition may also be treated with itraconazole (200 mg PO/IV QD). Cases refractory to azole therapy

ANSWERS

should be treated with IV amphotericin B. Keto-conazole is less effective than other azoles against candidal esophagitis.

91–C, 92–A

This patient is at risk for a number of opportunistic infections given his profound immunosuppression. Prophylaxis for a number of known infectious agents is initiated at different levels of immunosuppression. *Pneumocystis* prophylaxis is usually initiated at CD4 cell counts <200 cells/µL, and the most effective agent is trimethoprim-sulfamethoxazole (brand names of Bactrim or Septra). The most common secondary agents of PCP prophylaxis in the setting of a sulfa-allergy include dapsone, atovaquone, and aerosolized pentamidine. The latter agent is considered the least desirable

93–D, 94–B, 95–A, 96–C

The most common causes of acute pancreatitis in the U.S. are ethanol abuse, biliary tract disease, and idiopathic processes. Less common but important causes include medications, ERCP, hyperlipidemia, penetrating ulcers, pancreas divisum, infection, and abdominal trauma. Medications definitely associated with acute pancreatitis include azathioprine and 6-MP; thiazide diuretics and furosemide; sulfonamides, tetracycline, pentamidine and ddI; estrogens; and valproic acid. Other medications may be associated as well.

The diagnosis of acute pancreatitis is usually made on the basis of the clinical symptoms, elevated serum levels of pancreatic enzymes, and CT imaging. If gallstone pancreatitis is suspected, RUQ ultrasound can be helpful. If these studies

TABLE A92. Infectious Agents Requiring Primary Prophylaxis in HIV Disease

INFECTION	INDICATION	PREVENTIVE REGIMENS	
		FIRST CHOICE	SECOND CHOICE
Pneumocystis pneumonia (PCP)	CD4 count <200 cells/µL or oropharyngeal candidiasis	Trimethoprim-sulfamethoxazole (TMP-SMZ) 1 DS PO QD or 1 SS PO QD	1) Dapsone 50 mg PO BID or 100 mg PO QD; 2) Dapsone 50 mg PO QD + pyrimethamine 50 mg PO each week + leucovorin 25 mg PO each week; 3) Dapsone 200 mg + pyrimethamine 75 mg + leucovorin 25 mg PO each week; 4) Aerosolized pentamidine 300 mg nebulized each month; 5) Atovaquone 1500 mg PO QD; 6) TMP-SMZ 1 DS PO three times a week
Toxoplasma gondii	IgG positive for *Toxoplasma* and CD4 count <100 cells/µL	TMP-SMZ 1 DS PO QD	1) TMP-SMZ 1SS PO QD; 2) Dapsone 50 mg PO QD + pyrimethamine 50 mg PO each week + leucovorin 25 mg PO each week; 3) Atovaquone 1500 mg PO QD with or without pyrimethamine 25 mg PO QD + leucovorin 10 mg PO QD
Mycobacterium avium complex (MAC)	CD4 count <50 cells/µL	Azithromycin 1200 mg PO each week; or Clarithromycin 500 mg PO BID	1) Rifabutin 300 mg PO QD; 2) Azithromycin 1200 mg PO week + rifabutin 300 mg PO QD

alternative, as it is the least effective, is difficult to administer, and only protects against pulmonary, not extrapulmonary, *Pneumocystis*. Another infection requiring primary prophylaxis is MAC/MAI (*Mycobacterium avium complex* or *intercellulare*), for which either clarithromycin (500 mg PO BID) or azithromycin (1200 mg PO each week) is initiated at CD4 counts <50 cells/µL. *Toxoplasma gondii* infection requires primary prophylaxis with Bactrim (TMP-SMZ) at CD4 counts <100 cells/µL if the patient's toxoplasma IgG level is positive. An alternative agent to TMP-SMZ for *Toxoplasma* prophylaxis is dapsone plus pyrimethamine and leucovorin (see table). Other infectious agents do not require routine primary prophylaxis but each patient is evaluated individually for risks for particular infections, with particular vigilance in appropriately treating latent *M. tuberculosis* infection.

are unrevealing, ERCP with manometry can diagnose abnormalities in the pancreatic ducts and surrounding tissue.

Although most cases of acute pancreatitis are clinically mild, up to 25% of patients with the disease have a fulminant, complicated course, with pancreatic necrosis ± infection, large-volume fluid shifts, metabolic abnormalities, sepsis and ARDS, and multiorgan failure.

Several clinical scoring systems help to predict the risk of developing complicated disease. One of these, Ranson's score, measures *five* clinical signs on admission (age >55, WBC >16,000/mm^3, glucose >200 mg/dL, serum LDH >350 IU/L, AST >250 IU/L); and *six* signs during the initial 48 hours of hospitalization (10% decrease in hematocrit, increase in BUN >1.8 mmol/L, serum calcium <8 mg/dL, PaO$_2$ <60 mmHg, base deficit

>4 mmol/L, and fluid sequestration >6 liters). A score of three or greater at either time predicts a severe, necrotic course, with a sensitivity of 60% to 80%.

The management of clinically mild acute pancreatitis includes eliminating oral intake, giving intravenous fluids and analgesia, and discontinuing precipitating agents, such as ethanol or suspect medications. PO intake, starting with clear fluids, can be tried once pain has completely resolved. In the presence of cholangitis or jaundice, immediate ERCP should be considered, although this carries its own risk of morbidity.

If pancreatic necrosis is suspected, dynamic, helical CT scanning with IV contrast is the initial diagnostic procedure of choice. Areas of non-enhancement indicate necrosis, and are more apparent after the first 3 days of disease. With aggressive supportive care and intensive management of systemic complications, the mortality of uninfected necrotic pancreatitis is roughly 10%. The risk of infection is high, however, and the mortality of infected necrotic pancreatitis, with treatment, is 30%. On the basis of one controlled clinical trial showing that the antibiotic imipenem reduced the risk of infection, but not mortality, (Pederzoli P, Bassi C, Vesentini S, et al. Surg Gynecol Obstet 1993;176:480–483), this antibiotic is often recommended in necrotizing pancreatitis. CT-guided fine-needle aspiration of necrotic material is highly sensitive and specific for infection, and is indicated for patients who do not improve with aggressive supportive therapy and imipenem. Without urgent surgical debridement, infected necrotic pancreatitis is uniformly fatal.

97–B

N-acetylcysteine serves as a protective treatment for APAP overdose. Knowledge of its mechanism of action requires a review of the pathophysiology of APAP poisoning: Acetaminophen is extensively metabolized by the liver and is excreted in the urine, primarily as inactive glucuronate and sulfate conjugates. A small amount (4%) is metabolized by the cytochrome P450-dependent mixed-function oxidative enzymes to form a toxic metabolite, *N*-acetyl-*p*-benzoquinoneimine, which is responsible for the hepatocellular necrosis associated with acetaminophen overdose. When therapeutic doses of acetaminophen are given, this metabolite is quickly metabolized to a nontoxic derivative by glutathione and is excreted in the urine as conjugates of cysteine and mercapturic acid. When acetaminophen is

taken in toxic doses, the glucuronic acid or sulfate pathways become saturated and an increased amount of acetaminophen is metabolized by the cytochrome P450 system to form the toxic metabolite. Glutathione conjugation increases, but the amount of glutathione available is limited. Once the supply of glutathione becomes depleted, the toxic metabolite binds covalently and irreversibly to hepatic cellular protein macromolecules, causing cell damage and death. *N*-acetylcysteine protects the liver by restoring glutathione levels to allow increased metabolism of the remaining APAP.

98–B

The vitamin K-dependent clotting factors (depleted quickly in the face of hepatic injury) are factors II, VII, IX, and X.

99–E

Wilson's disease, also called hepatolenticular degeneration, is an autosomal recessive disorder of copper metabolism characterized by excessive accumulations of copper in the liver, central nervous system, kidneys, eyes, and other organs. Copper usually accumulates progressively in the liver, leading to ultimate liver failure. Ceruloplasmin is a serum copper-binding protein that is usually decreased in the diagnosis of Wilson's (although 5% of cases of Wilson's have normal ceruloplasmin levels).

100–C

Fulminant hepatic failure is seen very rarely as a presenting feature of hepatitis C infection. The other viruses are more likely to present as acute hepatic failure. Hepatitis D (the delta virus) is a small circular RNA virus which is replication-defective and can only propagate in the presence of hepatitis B virus. Superinfection by hepatitis D virus should be suspected in any patient with chronic hepatitis B whose liver function suddenly worsens.

101–B, 102–D

In analyzing the composition of ascitic fluid, the three most useful determinations are the albumin, differential cell count, and microbiological culture. If a malignancy is suspected, cytologic exam can also be useful. In a patient with new-onset ascites of unknown origin, the ascitic albumin is used to calculate the serum-ascites albumin gradient (SAAG), which is simply the

ANSWERS

serum albumin minus the ascitic albumin. A SAAG >1.1 is thought to reflect increased hydrostatic pressure in the portal circulation relative to the peritoneal cavity, and thus to indicate ascites due to portal hypertension or congestive heart failure. A SAAG <1.1 reflects a more exudative process, such as a malignancy, tuberculous or pyogenic peritonitis, or a pancreatic pseudocyst. The sensitivity of bacterial cultures for SBP depends on the culture medium used. The sensitivity of routine body-fluid culture bottles is 40% to 65%, whereas that of blood culture bottles inoculated at the bedside is 90%. The latter technique may not be acceptable in all clinical microbiology labs. The presumptive diagnosis of SBP can be made by cell count alone; a WBC count of at least 500, with at least 50% PMNs, or an absolute PMN count of 250, indicates the need for antibiotic therapy.

SBP is usually a monomicrobial infection. Empiric antibiotic therapy should cover the most commonly isolated pathogens: *Streptococcus pneumoniae* and *Escherichia coli*. Because *Enterococcus faecalis* can also cause SBP, ampicillin or piperacillin are sometimes added to the regimen. Many experts recommend avoiding aminoglycosides out of concern that their renal toxicity could lead to the hepatorenal syndrome. Oral fluoroquinolones or trimethoprim-sulfamethoxazole can be used to prevent recurrences of SBP.

103–D

Although the precise cause of hepatic encephalopathy is unknown, treatment consists of eliminating the causes of excess protein load and ammonia formation in the gut. Therapeutic measures include limiting dietary protein, purging the GI tract of blood if present, and controlling ammonia-production by intestinal flora. Lactulose decreases the amount of ammonia-producing gut flora. In addition, the digestion of lactulose by intestinal bacteria produces acidic waste products, which in turn convert ammonia (NH_3) to nonabsorbable ammonium (NH_4^+) ion. If lactulose alone is ineffective, oral Neomycin 0.5–1.0 gram q6–12h can be added to reduce the load of ammonia-producing bacteria in the intestine. In general, benzodiazepines should not be given to patients with hepatic encephalopathy. However, oxazepam, which is not hepatically metabolized, can be used in cases of extreme agitation.

104–C

Ascites refractory to diuretics can be treated with serial paracentesis, TIPS, or liver transplant.

Although TIPS is effective, complications include shunt stenosis, occlusion, and infection, as well as hepatic encephalopathy. TIPS is usually recommended as a temporizing measure while the patient awaits liver transplantation.

105–B, 106–D, 107–A, 108–C

Acute infection and malignancy have been essentially ruled out. The patient's history, physical examination, and serology are inconsistent with lupus. Of the vasculitic syndromes, Wegener's granulomatosis is unlikely given the lack of upper respiratory tract and lung findings, or of glomerulonephritis, and the negative cANCA; the patient's age and physical examination are inconsistent with both Takayasu's arteritis and giant cell arteritis; and Churg-Strauss syndrome is unlikely without asthma history, or eosinophilia. A positive pANCA titer can be seen in PAN, but is not required for the diagnosis. It is positive in up to three-fourths of patients with the related disease, microscopic polyangiitis. The constellation of symptoms in this patient, along with hypertension, leukocytosis, and anemia of chronic disease, are all consistent with PAN, which affects small and medium-sized arteries in the gut, kidneys, skin, peripheral nervous system, and occasionally coronary arteries and myocardium, while generally sparing the lung. In some cases, PAN has been associated with positive hepatitis B virus serologies.

The most sensitive and specific test for PAN is the presence of medium vessel vasculitis in a biopsy of tissue at a symptomatic site. Failing this, the diagnosis can be made by the demonstration of aneurysms in small and medium-sized vessels on mesenteric, renal, or hepatic angiography.

Untreated, PAN is a relentless disease, with a 5-year mortality rate of approximately 80%. Treatment with steroids ± cyclophosphamide decreases mortality greatly. PAN associated with hepatitis B infection has been reported to be successfully treated with steroids, plasma exchange, and antiviral therapy. Because the treatment of the primary vasculitis syndromes relies on high-dose steroids and cytotoxic agents, it is especially important to rule out infection before starting treatment.

109–C

Most patients in DKA have a fluid deficit of 4 to 5 liters, which should be replaced promptly, but not so rapidly as to cause pulmonary or cerebral edema. The usual recommendation is to give a liter of normal saline (NS) over the first hour of treatment, followed by NS at 300–500 mL/hour to a volume of 2 to 4 liters, followed by half-normal saline at 150–300 mL/hour. At least 3 to 4 liters should be replaced in the first 8 hours of therapy; replacing more than 5 liters in the same interval may increase the risk of pulmonary or cerebral edema. Once the blood glucose has fallen to 250 mg/dL, 5% dextrose can be added to the IV fluids.

Intravenous regular insulin both reduces hyperglycemia (and the resulting hyperosmolar diuresis), and reverses the metabolic acidosis of DKA (by removing ketones from the blood and reducing their production in the liver). A bolus of 0.15 units/kg is given immediately, followed by a constant drip at 0.10 units/kg/hour. It is essential to remember that the hyperglycemia of DKA will correct before the acidemia; therefore, the insulin drip should continue until the anion gap has closed, or else the patient will relapse into ketoacidosis. Once the anion gap has closed and the patient can tolerate PO intake, you can give 4–10 units of regular insulin SQ, along with some long-acting insulin, and turn off the insulin drip approximately 2 hours later.

Because managing a patient with DKA requires keeping track of and correcting many metabolic derangements, it is extremely helpful to use a flowsheet in drawing labs and recording results. Information should include the patient's presenting lab values, the doses and times of fluid and insulin administration, and a schedule of tests and results. Serum electrolytes should be checked (especially for K^+, osmolarity, glucose, and anion gap) every 2 hours, and magnesium and phosphate every 8 hours. Results of ECG, chest x-ray, and cultures should also be noted.

110–D

Although serum K^+ is initially elevated, this is due to the movement of K^+ out of cells under acidemic conditions. Polyuria and vomiting actually deplete the total body stores of K^+ in patients with DKA; as a result, the serum potassium tends to fall precipitously as the acidemia is treated, requiring close monitoring and frequent potassium repletion. In general, 10–20 mEq/hour of K^+ are given for serum values of 5 to 6. For serum values of <3.5, 40–80 mEq/hour can be given. As always, successful potassium repletion may depend on concurrent magnesium repletion.

111–C

If the serum glucose fails to decrease more than 10% in the first hour of therapy, the loading dose should be repeated.

112–D

In 20% to 25% of cases of DKA, the condition occurs without a clear precipitating event. Thirty to forty percent of cases are caused by infection, 20% by the new onset of diabetes, 15% to 20% by poor compliance with an established insulin regimen, and 10% to 15% by other medical events such as MI, pancreatitis, or CVA. It is therefore important to search for a concomitant illness in any patient presenting in DKA. However, the benefits of a CT in an otherwise asymptomatic patient are outweighed by costs.

113–C

Primary hypothyroidism is accompanied by decreases in free T_4 or free T_4 index, anemia and hyponatremia. Increases in TSH, serum cholesterol, serum triglycerides, LDH, ALT, and AST are also observed.

114–E

The distinctions between primary and secondary hypothyroidism are outlined in Table A114.

TABLE A114. The Primary Causes of Primary and Secondary Hypothyroidism

Primary Hypothyroidism
Hashimoto thyroiditis
Postpartum disease (transient)
Postirradiation disease
Subtotal thyroidectomy
Subacute thyroiditis (transient)
Antithyroid drugs [lithium, para-aminosalicylic acid (PAS), propylthiouracil (PTU), methimazole, iodide excess]
Iodide deficiency
Infiltrative disease (hemochromatosis, amyloidosis, scleroderma)
Biosynthetic defect, hereditary
Secondary Hypothyroidism
Pituitary macroadenoma
Empty sella syndrome
Infarction
Infiltrative disease (e.g., sarcoidosis)
Surgery or radiation-induced injury

115–B, 116–C

Subacute thyroiditis following a viral URI is a more transient form of thyroid injury. In this

ANSWERS

condition, the gland is very tender and enlarged, often asymmetrically. A brief period of hyperthyroidism may precede glandular hypofunction and subsequent hypothyroidism, but spontaneous remission and restoration of normal thyroid function is the rule. Pathologically, a granulomatous giant cell infiltrate and a marked reduction in iodine uptake characterize the condition. The clinical course ranges from weeks to a few months.

117–D

Primary hyperparathyroidism is the most common cause of hypercalcemia in ambulatory patients, whereas malignancy is responsible for most cases of hypercalcemia among hospitalized patients. Primary hyperparathyroidism results from excessive secretion of parathyroid hormone (PTH) and is most common in older women. Nearly 85% of the cases are due to an adenoma of a single gland; 15% to hyperplasia of all four glands; and 1% to parathyroid carcinoma. Many patients with this disorder are asymptomatic, with hypercalcemia being detected on routine laboratory screening. Serum PTH levels will also be elevated and parathyroidectomy is the only effective therapy.

118–A

The most common cause of hypercalcemia of malignancy is production by the tumor of PTHrP, or PTH-related peptide. PTHrP acts very similarly to PTH in activating bone resorption, leading to increased calcium levels. In 50% to 70% of patients with hypercalcemia and malignancy, elevated PTHrP is found; the peptide is most commonly elaborated by squamous cell carcinomas, renal cell carcinoma, and breast cancer. Tumor metastases to bone can also cause mobilization of calcium, but this latter mechanism for hypercalcemia in malignancy is more rare and associated most closely with multiple myeloma. Tumors can very rarely secrete authentic PTH or 1,25-dihydroxyvitamin D, leading to hypercalcemia. Mutations in the extracellular calcium-sensing receptor gene essential for regulation of calcium homeostasis is the genetic defect found in familial hypocalciuric hypercalcemia.

119–E

Hypercalcemia is most commonly associated with breast cancer, renal cell carcinoma, multiple myeloma, and squamous cell carcinomas of sites other than skin. Rare tumors associated with this disorder (but in a high percentage of cases) include small cell carcinoma of the ovary, HTLV-1

associated T cell leukemia, and high/intermediate grade non-Hodgkin lymphoma. There is no association between acute myelogenous leukemia and the hypercalcemia of malignancy.

120–C

A shortened QT interval is the most common electrocardiographic finding of hypercalcemia, largely secondary to the shortening of the ST segment. A prolonged PR interval can also be observed.

121–B

Primary adrenal failure is defined by primary adrenal gland failure, resulting in reduced cortisol stimulation to the pituitary gland, and increased production of ACTH by this gland. Secondary adrenal failure is defined by reduced ACTH production, usually secondary to hypothalamic or pituitary lesions, leading to reduced stimulation of the adrenal gland to produce cortisol. The ACTH level will thus be high in primary adrenal failure and low in secondary adrenal insufficiency.

122–A

One of the ways of distinguishing primary adrenal insufficiency from secondary (cortisol production inadequate due to insufficient pituitary ACTH secretion) or tertiary adrenal insufficiency is the prolonged ACTH stimulation test. ACTH is administered as a continuous infusion for 48 hours and plasma cortisol concentrations and urinary cortisol excretion are monitored. Cortisol secretion increases progressively in secondary or tertiary adrenal insufficiency, because the atrophic adrenal glands recover cortisol secretory capacity with ACTH stimulation. The adrenal glands in primary adrenal insufficiency are partially or completely destroyed and are already exposed to maximally stimulating levels of endogenous ACTH, so they do not respond to further ACTH stimulation.

123–D

Cortisol suppresses the production of eosinophils, so eosinophilia is often observed in the setting of adrenal insufficiency.

124–E

Primary adrenal insufficiency refers to primary disease of the adrenal glands, leading to deficiency of cortisol and often aldosterone, and resulting in elevated plasma ACTH levels. The most common causes of primary adrenal failure worldwide are autoimmune (idiopathic) destruction, often in the setting of polyglandular failure, and tuberculosis, through primary destruction of the adrenal gland. Rarer causes include fungal infections, adrenal hemorrhage, metastases to the adrenal gland, sarcoidosis, amyloidosis, HIV infection, congenital adrenal hyperplasia, and certain medications.

125–C

Although rare, lactic acidosis is the most serious complication of metformin. Its prevalence is increased in the presence of other risk factors for lactic acidosis, including renal insufficiency and intravenous administration of iodinated contrast, which may trigger alterations in renal function. Other side effects of metformin are usually gastrointestinal, with nausea, abdominal distention, and diarrhea among the most common. Asymptomatic subnormal levels of vitamin B_{12} in the presence of metformin administration have been reported, although resultant megaloblastic anemia is rare.

126–D

(See Case 35, Calculating Cholesterol.) Diabetes mellitus serves as a coronary heart disease equivalent; hence, patients with this condition should be considered for aggressive lipid lowering therapy to achieve an LDL goal of <100 mg/dL.

127–D

Hypertension in combination with diabetes mellitus accelerates the progression of nephropathy and the presymptomatic condition of clinical microalbuminuria. Thus, an aggressive approach to BP reduction (<130/80) has been recommended in diabetics, with ACE inhibitors and calcium channel blockers being on the forefront of recommended antihypertensive regimens secondary to their role in slowing renal failure in these patients. (See Case 50, Tired of Uremia.)

128–B

The major risk factors for type II diabetes are

- Family history of diabetes (i.e., parents or siblings with diabetes)
- Obesity (i.e., ≥20% over desired body weight or BMI ≥27 kg/m²)
- Habitual physical inactivity

- Race/ethnicity (e.g., increased risk in African-Americans, Hispanic-Americans, Native Americans, Asian-Americans, and Pacific Islanders)
- Previously identified elevated fasting plasma glucose
- Hypertension (≥140/90 in adults)
- HDL cholesterol ≤35 mg/dL
- Delivery of a baby weighing >9 lbs
- Polycystic ovary disease

129–B

Immediate clinical management of thyroid storm involves five goals: to inhibit hormone synthesis, to block hormone release, to prevent peripheral conversion of T_4 to T_3, to block the peripheral effects of thyroid hormone, and to provide general support, including management of atrial fibrillation if present. These patients should be taken to the ICU for close monitoring and the following management should be initiated:

1. Block synthesis: propylthiouracil, 150 mg PO/NG q6h.
2. Block release: potassium iodide (SSKI), 3 to 5 drops PO/NG q8h; Lugol's iodine solution, 30 drops per day in 3 to 4 divided doses by mouth (PO) or nasogastric (NG) tube; or sodium iodide, 1 gram slow IV drip every 8 to 12 hours.
3. Block peripheral effects:
   A. Block T_4 to T_3 conversion: hydrocortisone, 100 mg IV q8h; or dexamethasone, 2 mg PO/NG q6h
   B. Beta-blockade: propranolol 1–2 mg IV q15min PRN (to control atrial fibrillation as well)
4. Supportive care: Treat fever with antipyretics, heart failure with digoxin and diuretics. Gently hydrate.
5. Rule out infectious causes as a trigger (e.g., blood and urine cultures; CXR).

130–D

Granulocytopenia is the most serious side effect associated with methimazole, which occurs in 0.5% of patients. Baseline WBC should be obtained before starting therapy but monitoring of WBC is generally not helpful because granulocytopenia is an idiosyncratic reaction of sudden onset. Patients should be instructed to stop the medication immediately and notify their physician if they develop any symptoms of infection (e.g., pharyngitis, fever).

ANSWERS

131–C

Although both methimazole and propylthiouracil cross the placenta, have uncertain effects in pregnancy, and are classified as "Class D" in pregnant patients, PTU is generally considered safer than methimazole. Thus, PTU should be administered in women of child-bearing age for thyrotoxicosis. Radioactive iodine ablation is contraindicated during pregnancy, as fetal hypothyroidism can result.

132–B

Signs and symptoms of apathetic hyperthyroidism are few and subtle, and the initial appearance of disease may be single organ failure (e.g., heart failure), producing diagnostic confusion. The cause of apathetic hyperthyroidism is usually multinodular goiter rather than Graves disease, and the patients are therefore typically older (in their 70s or 80s), have small multinodular or nonpalpable goiters, and lack autoimmune ophthalmopathy. Cardiovascular symptoms, especially congestive heart failure and atrial fibrillation, are prominent, as might be expected from the advanced ages of the patients. Weight loss is significant, averaging 40 pounds in one study. Depressed mental function, ranging from a placid demeanor to frank coma, is usual, but this condition may alternate with tremor and hyperactivity. Although apathetic thyrotoxicosis usually occurs in the elderly, it has been reported in most age groups, including children.

133–B

The National Cholesterol Education Program (NCEP) recommendations regarding the treatment of patients with elevated LDL cholesterol depend on a given patient's LDL and number of risk factors for CAD. Risk factors include age; family history of early CAD in a first-degree relative; HDL cholesterol <35 mg/dL; hypertension regardless of treatment; diabetes mellitus regardless of treatment; and current cigarette smoking. Patients at low risk (fewer than two risk factors) with an LDL >160 mg/dL should receive diet therapy, while those with an LDL >190 mg/dL should receive drug therapy. In either case, the therapeutic target is an LDL <160 mg/dL. Patients at intermediate risk (two or more risk factors) and an LDL >130 mg/dL should receive diet therapy, while those with an LDL >160 mg/dL should receive drug therapy. In either case, the therapeutic target is an LDL <130 mg/dL. Patients with known CAD should maintain an LDL <100 mg/dL, and should receive drug therapy for an LDL >130 mg/dL. First-line therapy for modifying lipids includes HMG-CoA reductase inhibitors (statins), niacin, and, in some cases, bile acid–binding resins. Gemfibrozil, a fibric acid derivative, is used to lower triglycerides.

134–D

The Sixth Report of the Joint National Committee on the Detection, Evaluation, and Treatment of High Blood Pressure (referred to as JNC VI) describes in detail the thresholds for diagnosing and treating hypertension, and is an invaluable resource. It defines the upper limit of normal systolic and diastolic blood pressure as 140 and 90 mmHg, respectively. Measurement of blood pressure is notoriously variable, and the economic cost and potential side effects of lifelong pharmacologic therapy can be high. Unless they are symptomatic, patients found to have mildly (BP >140–159/90–99) or moderately (BP >160–179/100–109) elevated blood pressure should be treated for hypertension only after this finding is observed on three separate office visits over several months.

135–C

The best strategy for colon cancer screening remains unclear. It is important to remember that while FOBT and flexible sigmoidoscopy are probably complementary screening tests, a positive finding on either test should be followed by full colonoscopy (although there is debate about the need for colonoscopy after the finding of a single adenomatous polyp smaller than 10 mm).

136–E

In addition to the factors listed in the question, white race, age >50 years, history of endometrial cancer, fibrocystic disease with proliferative changes, and cancer in the contralateral breast confer an increased risk of developing breast cancer. A thorough menstrual history can uncover risk factors as well, such as menarche before age 12, menopause after age 50, nulliparity, or first pregnancy after age 35. Regardless of evidence, most guidelines also support screening for breast cancer among women younger than 50 or older than 65 who are at increased risk of developing disease.

137–B

Prior to the initiation of lipid-lowering therapy, any patient with hyperlipidemia should undergo clinical or laboratory assessment to rule out secondary causes of dyslipidemia. These secondary causes include diabetes, hypothyroidism, obstructive liver disease, chronic renal failure (usually accompanied by nephrotic syndrome), and drugs that increase LDL cholesterol and decrease HDL cholesterol (progesterones, anabolic steroids, and corticosteroids). Obesity is not a cause of secondary hyperlipidemia.

138–E

The category in which LDL goal is <100 mg/dL is the presence of CHD or "CHD risk equivalents." Diabetes qualifies as a CHD risk equivalent because it confers a high risk of new CHD within 10 years. In addition, diabetics who experience a MI have an unusually high death rate either immediately or in the long term, mandating more intensive risk factor modification.

139–D

Emerging risk factors for CHD include elevated apolipoprotein levels, elevated total plasma homocysteine levels, subclinical CAD determined by electron beam tomography (EBT), disorders of LDL subclass distribution (with an increased distribution in the small subclass regions), prothrombotic and proinflammatory factors, and impaired fasting glucose. Low HDL and peripheral arterial disease are known risk factors for CHD. Hypothyroidism is a secondary cause of hyperlipidemia. The evidence for chronic infections leading to an increased risk for CHD is still controversial, but the infectious agents thus far implicated (*Chlamydia pneumoniae*, *Helicobacter pylori*, CMV) do not include streptococci.

140–B

Statins (especially atorvastatin), nicotinic acid, and fibric acids (including gemfibrozil and clofibrate) all can decrease triglyceride levels to varying degrees, but bile acid sequestrants (such as cholestyramine) either do not change or can actually increase triglyceride levels.

141–B, 142–E

Table A142 shows the recommended and alternative treatment choices for latent TB infection in adults. Though a study in HIV patients (JAMA 2000;283:1445–50) showed the equivalency between 2 months of rifampin and PZA to 12 months of daily INH, recent reports of severe and fatal hepatotoxicity with this regimen (MMWR Morb Mortal Wkly Rep 2001;50:733–5) have unfavorably altered the recommendation for this regimen.

TABLE A142. Recommended Drug Regimens for Treatment of Latent TB in Adults

DRUG	INTERVAL DURATION	COMMENTS	RATING[a] HIV–	RATING[a] HIV+
Isoniazid	QD × 9 months	In HIV, can give with NRTIs, PIs, NNRTIs	A	A
	BIW × 9 months	DOT must be used with BIW therapy	B	B
Isoniazid[b]	QD × 6 months	Not indicated for HIV patients, those with fibrotic lesions on chest x-ray, or children	B	C
	BIW × 6 months	DOT must be used with BIW dosing	B	C
Rifampin[c]	QD × 4 months	For persons who cannot tolerate PZA For persons who are contacts of patients with INH-R, rifampin-S TB who cannot tolerate PZA	B	B
Rifampin[c] plus PZA	QD × 2 months	Also for patients who are contacts of patients with INH-R, rifampin-S TB In HIV patients, rifampin generally not used with PIs or NNRTIs; can substitute rifabutin[d]	C	C

[a]Strength of recommendation: A = preferred; B = acceptable alternative; C = offer when A and B cannot be given.
[b]Children under 18 years of age should receive 9-month regimens.
[c]Pregnant women should use INH regimens, not rifampin-based regimen.
[d]Rifabutin should not be used with hard-gel saquinavir or delavirdine. Dose adjustment of rifabutin may be necessary with other HAART agents.

143–C, 144–D

Hepatitis is the most severe toxic effect of INH. Peripheral neuropathy can occur in patients with INH, as the drug does interfere with pyridoxine

ANSWERS

metabolism, so vitamin B_6 should be coadminis-tered in patients prone to neuropathy.

145–E, 146–C, 147–B, 148–B

This patient has community-acquired pneumococ-cal meningitis secondary to otitis media and pansi-nusitis. The organism is intermediately resistant to penicillin. Although the mechanisms of penicillin re-sistance and macrolide resistance in *Streptococcus pneumoniae* differ, multiple-antibiotic resistance is common among penicillin-resistant strains.

The standard microbiologic workup for sus-pected meningitis includes sending the CSF for smear, cell count and differential, protein, glu-cose, and culture for bacteria, AFB, and fungus. In the proper clinical setting, sending CSF for HSV PCR would also be appropriate. If a patient is at risk for cryptococcal meningitis, the serum crypto-coccal antigen test is 95% sensitive for infection; the CSF cryptococcal antigen test is 100% sensi-tive, and the titer can be useful in following the success of treatment in HIV-infected patients.

Although you know from the CSF smear and culture that the patient has penicillin-resistant pneumococcal meningitis, that information was unavailable when you initiated antibiotic treat-ment. Community-acquired bacterial meningitis in an adult (18 to 50 years old) is most commonly caused by *Streptococcus pneumoniae* or *Neisseria meningitides.* Standard empiric therapy includes cefotaxime, 2 grams IV q6h, or ceftriaxone, 2 grams IV q12h. In areas with penicillin-resistant pneumo-coccus, vancomycin, 15 mg/kg q8h, should also be given. Given the increasing incidence of pneumo-coccal penicillin resistance worldwide, many experts recommend the empiric use of vancomycin in all cases of suspected invasive pneumococcal disease until sensitivities are known. In adults over 50 years of age, *Listeria monocytogenes* can also cause meningitis, so ampicillin, 2 grams IV q4h, should be added empirically. Aminoglycosides IV, such as gentamicin, penetrate the CSF very poorly. Fluoroquinolones such as ciprofloxacin are not standard first-line antibiotics in bacterial meningi-tis. Although many reported histories of penicillin allergy are spurious, a patient who reports symp-toms of anaphylaxis to penicillin should not receive a β-lactam antibiotic without skin testing. A full discussion of the treatment of pneumococ-cal meningitis in the β-lactam-allergic patient is beyond the scope of this text. Nevertheless, some experts recommend that rifampin be added to vancomycin, given the variable penetration of the latter drug into the CSF, while issues surrounding a potential β-lactam allergy are being resolved.

149–E

Risk factors such as nasal polyps, deviated nasal septum, trauma, foreign bodies, allergic rhinitis, and rapid changes in altitude can predispose to acute sinusitis. Although eczema suggests atopy, it is not enough to predispose a patient to sinusitis.

150–A

Ancillary treatment in sinusitis is directed at facil-itating drainage of the sinus and nasal passages and relieving sneezing, coughing, and systemic symptoms. Decongestants are vasoconstrictors that reduce the thickness of the nasal mucosa. Oral decongestants include pseudoephedrine, phenylpropanolamine, and phenylephrine, and offer the theoretical advantage over topical decongestants of reducing congestion in deeper tissues. Nasal sprays, such as phenylephrine hydrochloride and oxymetazoline hydrochloride, may provide immediate symptomatic relief. How-ever, prolonged use of topical agents may cause rebound vasodilation, irritation, and reactive hyperemia. Expectorants, such as guaifenesin, have been used on theoretical grounds to thin secretions and aid drainage, although their effi-cacy is still under study. Saline lavage of the nasal cavities, steam inhalation, and drinking plenty of water can also help clear secretions.

Antihistamines are generally not recom-mended for acute sinusitis because of concerns of drying of mucous membranes and impeding clearance of secretions. The exception is sinusitis in allergic patients during the allergy season. Topical or systemic steroids have been reported to reduce local sinus osteal inflammation, but their routine use in all patients with sinusitis does not appear warranted, except in patients with allergic or chronic sinusitis.

151–C

Amoxicillin is considered first-line therapy for acute bacterial sinusitis, with trimethoprim-sulfamethoxazole for penicillin-allergic patients. Secondary lines of treatment include amoxicillin-clavulanate (Augmentin), second- and third-generation oral cephalosporins, macrolides, and fluoroquinolones. However, the latter options are probably too broad-spectrum for this condition. Physicians must keep in mind that bacterial sinusitis complicates only 0.5% to 5.0% of the millions of cases of acute viral URIs and that 30% to 50% of aspirates show no likely pathogen. Hence, the role of antibiotics in uncomplicated bacterial sinusitis has been questioned. A recent study (van Buchem et al. Lancet 1997;349:683–68) showed that antibiotics offered no therapeutic advantage over symptomatic treatment alone, which led the investigators to conclude that in newly presenting patients with maxillary sinusitis, initial management could be limited to symptomatic treatment. In clinical trials, the placebo response rate is high (>60%) and is enhanced by decongestant treatment.

152–D

Sinusitis is the primary source of infection in approximately two-thirds of patients with intracranial abscesses.

153–E, 154–E, 155–C, 156–D

Group A beta-hemolytic streptococcal (GABHS) pharyngitis is usually a self-limited disease, resolving locally within 7 days. The most important reasons for treatment are to prevent serious local complications, particularly peritonsillar abscess formation, and to prevent systemic complications, such as postinfectious glomerulonephritis and rheumatic fever. Bacteriologic throat culture is the most reliable test for GABHS. Because the rapid streptococcal antigen test fails to detect 15% to 20% of cases, it cannot be used to rule out infection. Treating for GABHS presumptively, treating on the basis of a positive antigen test used to confirm a clinical suspicion, or waiting for culture-directed therapy before treating are three reasonable therapeutic approaches. It is important to remember that treatment for GABHS is effective at preventing rheumatic fever when started within 1 week of the onset of symptoms.

With penicillin, the symptoms of GABHS pharyngitis should resolve within 72 hours of beginning treatment. Acceptable alternatives to penicillin include amoxicillin, cephalexin, cefuroxime, clindamycin, and macrolides. Concern over the acquisition of cephalosporin-resistance by endogenous flora has prompted some reviewers to discourage the treatment of pharyngitis with cephalosporins when alternatives exist.

Some possible reasons for the failure of GABHS pharyngitis to improve after 72 hours of penicillin therapy include: the development of a peritonsillar abscess; concurrent viral infection; nonadherence to treatment; or β-lactam production by oral anaerobes. The possibility of a deep-space infection, such as an abscess, requires prompt evaluation.

Because of the increased incidence of penicillin-resistant *Neisseria gonorrhoeae,* ceftriaxone is the treatment of choice for gonococcal pharyngitis.

Doxycycline or azithromycin should be added to cover *Chlamydia trachomatis,* which is often present as well.

157–D

The differential diagnosis for thrombocytopenia is given in Table A157. The diagnosis of ITP is based principally on the history, physical examination, complete blood count, and examination of the peripheral smear, which should exclude other causes of thrombocytopenia. Further diagnostic studies, such as bone marrow aspiration, are generally not indicated in the routine workup of patients with suspected ITP, assuming that the history, physical examination, and blood counts are compatible with the diagnosis. Patients with risk factors for HIV infection should be tested for HIV antibody, as HIV is an associated condition. I.T. has a history consistent with acute ITP, as she has never experienced any bleeding problems previously, even in a previous operation, and she has an isolated thrombocytopenia with normal red blood cell morphology and white blood cell morphology on blood smear. There is no evidence for a microangiopathic process (e.g., TTP or DIC) or platelet satellitism on her blood smear.

TABLE A157. Pathophysiologic Classification of Thrombocytopenia

Artifactual thrombocytopenia
Platelet clumping caused by anticoagulant-dependent immunoglobulin (pseudothrombocytopenia)
Platelet satellitism
Giant platelets

Decreased platelet production
Hypoplasia of megakaryocytes
Ineffective thrombopoiesis
Disorders of thrombopoietic control
Hereditary thrombocytopenias

Increased platelet destruction
Caused by immunologic processes
Autoimmune
  Idiopathic
  Secondary: infections, pregnancy, collagen vascular disorders, lymphoproliferative disorders, drugs, miscellaneous
Alloimmune
  Neonatal thrombocytopenia
  Post-transfusion purpura

Caused by nonimmunologic processes
Thrombotic microangiopathies
  Disseminated intravascular coagulation
  Thrombotic thrombocytopenic purpura
  Hemolytic-uremic syndrome
Platelet damage by abnormal vascular surfaces
Miscellaneous
  Infection
  Massive blood transfusions

Abnormal platelet distribution or pooling
  Disorders of the spleen (neoplastic, congestive, infiltrative, infectious, of unknown cause)
  Hypothermia
  Dilution of platelets with massive transfusions

ANSWERS

158–D

Although not routinely measured in the diagnosis of this disease, antiplatelet antibodies are often elevated (85% to 90%) in ITP, as they are instrumental for the pathophysiology of this condition. Evidence is now convincing that the syndrome of ITP is caused by platelet-specific autoantibodies that bind to autologous platelets which are then rapidly cleared from the circulation by the mononuclear phagocyte system. The ITP antibody does not fix complement in vitro when tested by the usual techniques, but activation of components of complement on the platelet surface may be demonstrated. LDH, fibrinogen, and PT/PTT are often elevated in TTP, as is creatinine if renal abnormalities exist, but not in ITP.

159–C

Immune-mediated thrombocytopenia can either be idiopathic (primary) or secondary.

- Idiopathic (primary)
- Secondary
  - Infections
  - Collagen vascular diseases (most commonly SLE)
  - Lymphoproliferative disorders
  - Solid tumors
  - Drugs
  - Medications (quinine/quinidine, sulfonamides, heparin, aspirin, and ethanol)
  - Miscellaneous (including HIV)

I.T. was using quinine sulfate for leg cramps, which may have been the inciting factor for her condition.

160–E

Treatment is indicated routinely in patients with platelet counts <20,000 and those with counts >30,000 only if significant mucous membrane bleeding is present (or risk factors for bleeding, such as hypertension, peptic ulcer disease, or a vigorous lifestyle, exist). In addition, hospitalization is appropriate for patients with platelet counts <20,000 who have significant mucous membrane bleeding, or in any patient with severe, life-threatening bleeding for conventional critical care measures and ITP treatment. Initial treatment for ITP includes glucocorticoid therapy (high-dose parenteral at first) and IVIg. Platelet transfusions are usually not helpful in ITP, as the antiplatelet antibodies will attack the new infused platelets, and will indeed be stimulated by platelet infusion; however, platelet transfusions can be used as a temporizing measure in setting of brisk bleeding or prior to surgery.

Splenectomy should not be performed as initial therapy in patients with minor symptoms, but is often appropriate in a patient who has had major bleeding (e.g., severe epistaxis, menorrhagia), or if platelet counts remain below 30,000 after 4 to 6 weeks of medical treatment. If an elective splenectomy is planned, appropriate preoperative therapy includes prophylactic IVIg or oral glucocorticoid therapy for patients with platelet counts <20,000.

When bleeding persists after primary treatment and splenectomy, and/or the platelet count remains below 30,000, further therapy may be indicated. The most commonly recommended options include more IVIg, routine glucocorticoids, and searching for and removing accessory spleens. Plasmapheresis is the modality of choice for TTP, not ITP.

161–E, 162–B, 163–E, 164–C

Several complications of acute leukemia are commonly encountered and should be screened for. Elevated levels of serum urate, found in up to 50% of patients, can precipitate in the kidney and cause renal failure, particularly after chemotherapy is started. Prophylaxis with allopurinol and bicarbonate can help prevent this process. This patient's anemia is secondary to the leukemia and possibly bleeding; iron studies are unnecessary at this point. Liver dysfunction may require adjustments in chemotherapy dosing. Disseminated intravascular coagulation (DIC), ranging from lab abnormalities (prolonged PT, decreased fibrinogen, elevated FSP) to life-threatening hemorrhage, can be seen, particularly in M3, or acute promyelocytic, leukemia. Treatment includes the administration of platelets, fibrinogen (using via cryoprecipitate), coagulation factors (using fresh frozen plasma), and in cases of active bleeding, heparin. Patients with extremely elevated numbers of circulating blasts are at risk for leukostasis, leading to ischemia or hemorrhage, and require immediate leukapheresis and chemotherapy. Finally, many patients with acute leukemia will be neutropenic and at risk for rapidly life-threatening infections. It is essential to determine the patient's absolute neutrophil count each day. Fever is very common among leukemic patients, whether or not an infection can be found. Nevertheless, febrile neutropenia is an oncologic emergency and requires immediate pan-culture and empiric antibiotic coverage for gram-positive and nosocomial gram-negative organisms.

165–B

The laboratory abnormalities associated with iron deficiency anemia change in stages. As iron stores are depleted, the ferritin level falls and the TIBC rises, indicating depleted stores and a high potential to bind iron if iron is present. The serum iron then falls, and erythrocytes become microcytic. A low ferritin level is therefore a more sensitive test for iron deficiency anemia than a low MCV, because the MCV can be normal early in the process.

166–A

The best treatment for iron deficiency anemia is oral iron supplementation, which should continue for 3 to 6 months after correction of the anemia, to replete iron stores. Intravenous iron can be substituted if a patient cannot tolerate or absorb oral iron. Because it can cause anaphylaxis, intravenous iron therapy requires a test dose and hemodynamic monitoring, with resuscitation equipment immediately available. Iron deficiency anemia should *always* prompt an evaluation for sources of blood loss, particularly from the GI tract.

167–D

Although anemia of chronic disease, another commonly encountered syndrome, is occasionally caused by insufficient erythropoietin production due to chronic renal failure, it is usually caused by the inappropriate sequestration of iron stores in the reticuloendothelial system during chronic illness. Typical underlying diseases include liver disease, chronic inflammation or infection, and neoplasms. Laboratory evidence of ACD shows both decreased serum iron, and decreased TIBC (i.e., decreased potential to store iron, because so much is already sequestered). The ferritin level, reticulocyte count, and peripheral smear are normal.

168–C

Based on his history and hematologic workup, this patient has anemia of chronic disease, most likely due to chronic HCV infection. There is no evidence of iron deficiency or renal failure. Injection drug use carries a risk of clostridial infections, which can cause life-threatening necrotizing fasciitis and hemolysis. This patient has neither the clinical picture nor the lab abnormalities associated with such an infection.

169–D

A review of TTP and HUS cases presenting at UCSF over a decade (Blood 1992;80:1890–5) revealed that, at the time of diagnosis, the lactate dehydrogenase (LDH) level was elevated in 98% of cases, with a median value of 1,208 U/L. Indeed, some clinicians have advocated that an elevated LDH be added to the classic diagnostic pentad of TTP. Coagulation parameters, fibrinogen, and fibrin split products are rarely abnormal in TTP/HUS syndromes.

170–B

It is estimated that about 90% of children with HUS have some evidence of vero cytotoxin-producing *E. coli* (VTEC) infection and that the serotype 0157:H7 can be demonstrated in two-thirds by culture, by the detection of free verotoxin in the feces, or both. Intriguingly, a recent prospective cohort study (Wong CS, Jelacic S, Habeeb RL, et al. N Engl J Med 2000;342:1930–1936) revealed that antibiotic treatment of children with *E. coli* O157:H7 infection increases the risk of developing HUS, as compared with symptomatic treatment alone.

171–C

TTP is a medical emergency and mandates the initiation of plasmapheresis as soon as possible. While the latter is being arranged, patients can be maintained on infusions of fresh frozen plasma. Patients who are refractory to plasmapheresis may respond to cryosupernatant plasma therapy, vincristine, intravenous immunoglobulin, prostacyclin, or splenectomy. The benefits of corticosteroids or antiplatelet drugs are uncertain, although steroid therapy is the mainstay of treatment in the syndrome of ITP.

172–A

TTP is associated with HIV infection, explaining the increase in cases of TTP seen in the era of the HIV epidemic.

173–D, 174–C

The history of risk behaviors in this patient and laboratory evaluation point to a diagnosis of acute antiretroviral syndrome from an initial

ANSWERS

exposure to human immunodeficiency virus (HIV). Acute HIV infection can have a number of clinical manifestations but usually results in a mononucleosis-like illness of rapid onset and varying severity, with approximately 80% of patients manifesting some symptoms during seroconversion (Table A174).

TABLE A174. The Most Common Signs, Symptoms, and Laboratory Values and Their Frequency with Primary HIV Infection

SIGNS, SYMPTOMS, LABORATORY VALUES	FREQUENCY (%)
Fevers	>90
Fatigue	>90
Rash	>70
Headache	32–70
Lymphadenopathy	40–70
Pharyngitis	50–70
Myalgias, arthralgias	50–70
Nausea, vomiting, or diarrhea	30–60
Night sweats	50
Oral ulcers	10–20
Genital ulcers	5–15
Thrombocytopenia	45
Leukopenia	40
Elevated hepatic enzymes	21

Among the most suggestive signs and symptoms are fever, skin and mucosal lesions, lymphadenopathies, and headache associated with retro-orbital pain. A maculopapular rash occurs at the onset of primary HIV infection in 30% to 50% or more of patients. The rash is nonpruritic and consists of macular or maculopapular lesions predominantly on the trunk, neck, and face. The rash is also frequently associated with mucocutaneous oral, genital, and anal ulcers and resolves spontaneously within 2 weeks. In most cases, the acute antiretroviral syndrome is self-limited, with a mean duration of 2 to 3 weeks.

Seroconversion is marked by the appearance of anti-HIV-specific antibodies in plasma and usually occurs 5 to 10 days after the acute antiretroviral syndrome and 3 to 8 weeks after infection. Following HIV infection, the sequence of markers to identify infection in their chronologic order of appearance in serum are viral RNA, p24 antigen (a viral core protein encoded by the HIV *gag* gene), and anti-HIV antibody. About 2 weeks after infection, viremia is thought to increase exponentially and then decline to a steady-state level as the humoral and cell-mediated immune responses control HIV replication (Figure A174). This time interval, the serologic "window period," is characterized by seronegativity, usually detectable p24 antigenemia, high viremia (as measured by RNA), and variable CD4 lymphocyte levels. Detection of specific antibody to HIV signals the end of the window period and labels the individual as seropositive.

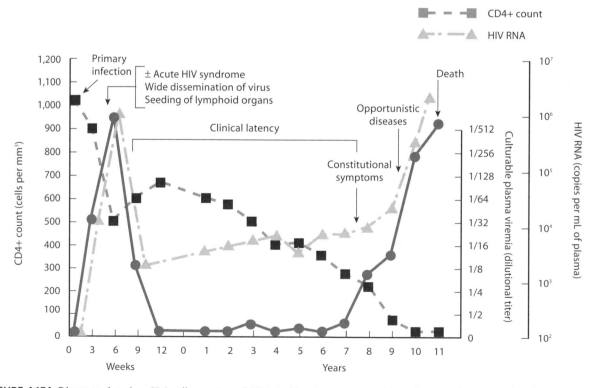

FIGURE A174 Diagram showing CD4 cell counts and HIV viral load, as measured by culture and HIV-RNA levels, throughout the natural course of HIV infection. (Illustration by Shawn Girsberger Graphic Design.)

175–A

Support for the concept of treatment during primary HIV infection comes from recent observations that show that HIV may be more vulnerable to antiretroviral therapy during primary infection. The reasons for treatment efficacy include:

- The immune system remains relatively intact although the rate of loss of CD4 cells may be increasing with concomitant primary HIV infection.
- HIV virus–specific cytotoxic T cells may be preserved through treatment of acute HIV infection (Rosenberg et al. Nature 2000;407:523–6).
- Newly infected persons tend to have a relatively homogeneous swarm of viruses, whereas persons with long-term infection have a diverse swarm of viruses. The low degree of diversity among viral isolates soon after initial infection suggests that there are relatively few resistant isolates, enhancing the efficacy of treatment during primary HIV infection.

Essentially, it is thought that augmentation of the initial immune response to HIV with effective antiretroviral medications may lead to enhanced control of HIV during primary HIV infection. Effective antiviral treatment during primary infection might lower the viral load set point, suppress subsequent viral replication, and lead to a prolonged period of asymptomatic disease. However, given the side effect profiles of these medications and the long-term complications, this decision must be made after fully informing the patient about the risks and benefits of initial therapy, and in consultation with a provider specialized in treating HIV.

176–D

Although the mechanism is not known, administering amoxicillin or penicillin in the setting of an acute infectious mononucleosis syndrome with EBV results in an almost 100% chance of developing a diffuse maculopapular rash.

177–C

The antibodies most commonly studied for the detection of a recent streptococcal infection are antistreptolysin O (ASO), antistreptokinase, antihyaluronidase, antideoxyribonuclease B, and antinicotinamide-dinucleotidase. The most commonly used test is the ASO, and an elevated ASO titer above 200 units is found in 90% of patients with pharyngeal infection. In the diagnosis of poststreptococcal glomerulonephritis, a rise in titer is more specific than the absolute level of a titer, but ASO titers are rarely obtained in the setting of acute infection. This patient's clinical picture, preceding syndrome of untreated pharyngitis, and elevated ASO titer are all highly suggestive of a poststreptococcal glomerulonephritis.

178–E, 179–D

Poststreptococcal glomerulonephritis (PSGN) occurs only after infection with certain nephritogenic strains of Group A beta-hemolytic streptococci, usually following an episode of pharyngitis or skin infection. PSGN is an immune complex disease in its acute phase and is characterized by the formation of antibodies against streptococcal antigens and the localization of immune complexes with complement in the kidney. Treatment is generally supportive, with spontaneous resolution of the syndrome 7 to 10 days after presentation. However, long-term hypertension or even renal insufficiency can develop as a result of PSGN.

180–B

The common name for IgA nephropathy is Berger's disease, which is now recognized as the most frequent form of idiopathic glomerulonephritis worldwide. This disease has a male predominance, with a peak occurrence in the second to third decades of life, and can progress to ESRD.

181–A, 182–B, 183–C

This patient is suffering from an attack of gout. Gout is a chronic disease associated with abnormally high levels of uric acid, and characterized in its early phases by acute flares of (usually) monoarthritis, and in its later phases by the presence of chronic urate crystal deposits (tophi) in joints and skin, and in the renal medulla and pyramids (uric acid renal stones). The overproduction or underexcretion of uric acid that is associated with gout can be either primary (idiopathic) or due to underlying conditions. Purine-rich foods, solid or liquid tumors, low-dose aspirin, and cytotoxic agents lead to urate overproduction, whereas renal tubular disease and certain drugs such as probenecid and thiazide diuretics impair uric acid clearance. Alcohol does both. Because serum urate levels fluctuate during gout flares, their measurement does not help in diagnosis.

Gout flares respond promptly to NSAIDs and oral or intra-articular steroids. Colchicine can also

ANSWERS

be used, but is associated with GI side effects. It is important to rule out a coexisting joint infection before treating gouty arthritis with steroids.

Avoiding alcohol, shellfish, and thiazide diuretics can prevent gout flares. When behavior modification is impossible or unsuccessful, daily colchicine helps prevent recurrence. If the above methods fail, a 24-hour urine collection can be performed to determine whether the patient is an urate overproducer or underexcretor. Allopurinol, which decreases urate production, or uricosuric agents such as probenecid or sulfinpyrazone, which increase urate excretion by blocking its reabsorption in the kidney, can be prescribed accordingly. Because abrupt changes in serum urate levels can precipitate a gout flare, neither allopurinol nor uricosuric agents should be started without a concomitant agent, such as colchicine, an NSAID, or oral steroid, to prevent an acute attack.

184–B

This is diagnostic of pseudogout, another type of acute monoarthritis caused by the deposition of crystals, in this case calcium pyrophosphate. Pseudogout is often associated with an underlying metabolic disorder. Treatment involves NSAIDs and/or intra-articular steroids, as well as treatment of the underlying disorder.

185–D

The most likely diagnosis in this patient is systemic lupus erythematosus (SLE). SLE is an inflammatory autoimmune disorder that may affect multiple organ systems and is nine times more common in women than men, four times more common in blacks than whites, and usually manifests in people between the ages of 15 and 45. Hence, this patient is in a relatively high-risk group for this disorder. Discoid lupus erythematosus manifests as the typical discoid rash (one example of which is shown above) without systemic symptoms; another form of lupus in which rash predominates is subacute cutaneous lupus. The most common presenting symptoms (in order of frequency) are musculoskeletal (usually fleeting or sustained polyarthritis, predominantly of the metacarpophalangeal, interphalangeal, and wrist joints); constitutional symptoms, such as malaise, fatigue, low-grade fevers (sometimes high fever), lymphadenopathy, and weight loss; rashes, either erythema or the typical raised rash involving the shawl area, the extensor surfaces of the upper arms, the finger pulps and periungual

areas (the classic malar "butterfly" rash occurs only in a minority of patients); hair loss; serositis; nondescript abdominal pain; or an incidental finding of a test abnormality, such as a hematologic problem. Myelopathy, myocarditis, pulmonary hypertension, acute lupus pneumonitis, pulmonary fibrosis, lupus profundus, and acute psychosis are rare initial symptoms of lupus.

186–B, 187–C, 188–C

The American College of Rheumatology has devised 11 diagnostic criteria for SLE. When a patient has four of the criteria in Table A188, she is said to have SLE. However, SLE is largely a clinical diagnosis and the following criteria should not be used wholly to exclude or confirm the diagnosis.

TABLE A188. 1997 Update of the 1982 American College of Rheumatology Classification Criteria for SLE

ITEM	DEFINITION
Malar rash	Fixed erythema over malar areas, sparing nasolabial folds
Discoid rash	Erythematous raised patches with keratotic scaling and follicular plugging
Photosensitivity	Skin rash after exposure to sunlight, history or physical exam
Oral ulcers	Oral or nasopharyngeal, painless, by physical exam
Nonerosive arthritis	Tenderness, swelling, effusion in two or more peripheral joints
Pleuritis or pericarditis	Convincing history or physical exam or ECG or other evidence
Renal disorder	>0.5g/d or 3+ protein uria or cellular casts
Seizures, psychosis	Not due to drugs, metabolic derangement, etc.
Hematologic disorder	Hemolytic anemia or leukopenia (<4000 twice) or lymphopenia (<1500 twice) or thrombocytopenia (<100,000) without other causes
Immunologic disorder	Anti-dsDNA or anti-Sm or antiphospholipid antibodies (anticardiolipin, lupus anticoagulant, or false-positive test for syphilis)
Positive ANA	Not drug induced

189–B

The patient has peripheral edema, proteinuria of greater than 3.5 grams/liter over 24 hours, and hypoalbuminemia, a triad of findings that defines the nephrotic syndrome. Underlying the nephrotic syndrome is a disruption in the glomerular physiology responsible for regulating protein retention, leading to excessive urinary protein excretion. The peripheral edema experienced by patients with the nephrotic syndrome may progress to pulmonary edema, and is thought to result either from a loss of oncotic pressure or a primary renal defect causing salt and water retention. This patient's labs show no evidence of chronic liver disease; her hepatitis serologies indicate resolved HBV infection, with resulting immunity.

190–D, 191–D

The pattern of glomerulonephropathy seen on renal biopsy can be helpful in: diagnosing either systemic or intrinsic renal causes of the nephrotic syndrome; suggesting the appropriate therapy; and estimating prognosis. The four major glomerulonephropathies associated with the nephrotic syndrome are minimal-change disease (MCD), focal segmental glomerulosclerosis (FSGS), membranous nephropathy, and membranoproliferative glomerulonephropathy (MPGN). All can be, and usually are, idiopathic, although certain types are associated with systemic illnesses. A partial list of the extrarenal causes of nephrotic syndrome includes: medical therapy with NSAIDs, gold, or penicillamine; Hodgkin's disease and certain carcinomas; HIV infection; bacterial endocarditis; heroin use; hepatitis B and C; and allergies and certain autoimmune diseases. Diabetic nephropathy and amyloidosis frequently cause the nephrotic syndrome as well. The degree and rapidity of chronic renal failure varies with the type of glomerulonephropathy underlying the nephrotic syndrome. In addition, the response of the nephrotic syndrome to therapy with steroids and cytotoxic agents varies considerably with the type of glomerolonephropathy involved. Any patient with new-onset nephrotic syndrome deserves a renal consultation.

This patient's past medical history raises the possibility of underlying HIV infection; both renal biopsy and HIV serology should be considered. Cases of HIV nephropathy with nephrotic syndrome have responded to high doses of prednisone and, more recently, highly active antiretroviral therapy. If you suspected underlying SLE, determining the ANA, dsDNA, and serum complement levels would be useful. If the urine salicylate test is positive, a follow-up serum and urine protein electrophoresis would be indicated to investigate the possibility of a plasma cell disorder or amyloidosis.

192–C

The inappropriate excretion of proteins caused by the nephrotic syndrome has numerous clinical consequences besides edema. The loss of antithrombin III, protein C, and protein S, and increased activation of platelets, can lead to venous and arterial hypercoagulability, particularly if the serum albumin falls to below 2 g/dL. Coumadin is indicated if DVT, pulmonary embolism, or arterial thrombi are diagnosed. Renal vein thrombosis is of particular concern, and requires indefinite anticoagulation. ACE inhibitors retard the development of nephrotic syndrome in diabetic nephropathy. The loss of oncotic pressure associated with the nephrotic syndrome seems to trigger increased lipoprotein synthesis, which may benefit from therapy with HMG-CoA reductase inhibitors. Edema can be treated with sodium restriction and loop diuretics. Intravenous albumin is of no use in either increasing oncotic pressure or compensating for protein malnutrition.

193–B

The most likely diagnosis is rheumatoid arthritis (RA) given the constellation of findings, including morning stiffness, swelling of the wrist joints, positive rheumatoid factor and the inflammatory nature of the aspirated fluid. The range of WBC in RA joints is usually 5000–20,000 compared with 50,000–300,000 in septic arthritis. Neutrophil percentage in RA is usually 50% to 70%, glucose levels are 10% to 25% less than serum, protein levels are >3.0 g/dL, and cultures are negative. The diagnosis of RA is a clinical one and requires that four of the seven criteria in Table A193 be fulfilled.

TABLE A193. Classification Criteria for Rheumatoid Arthritis

Morning stiffness for ≥1 hour
Swelling (soft tissue) of three or more joints
Swelling (soft tissue) of hand joints (PIP, MCP, or wrist)
Symmetrical swelling (soft tissue)
Subcutaneous nodules
Serum rheumatoid factor
Erosions and/or periarticular osteopenia in hand or wrist joints seen on radiograph

Note: Criteria 1 through 4 must have been continuous for 6 weeks or longer. Criteria 2 through 5 must be observed by a physician.

The frequently diagnosed syndrome of fibromyalgia, usually affects women between 25 and 50 years old, and is characterized by sometimes debilitating, diffuse musculoskeletal pain. The areas most commonly affected include the posterior muscles of the neck and scapula, the soft tissues lateral to the thoracic and lumbar spine, and the sacroiliac joint. Patients with this

ANSWERS

syndrome often have accompanying emotional or physical stress, depression, fatigue, and sleep disturbances. Other common symptoms include fatigue, sensation of swelling in the hands and feet, morning stiffness, headaches, and paresthesias. Cold weather seems to precipitate the syndrome in these patients. The examiner can elicit the pain by applying pressure over certain spots in the areas described above, called "trigger points." The cause is uncertain, but seems to be related to serotonin depletion and other physiologic responses to sleep disturbances. Treatment is often multidisciplinary, involving sleep conditioning, pain control, aerobic exercise, stress reduction, psychotherapy, and antidepressants.

194–E

Genetic susceptibility to RA has been demonstrated: the disease clusters in families and is more concordant in monozygotic (30%) than dizygotic (5%) twins. Among Caucasians of Western European origin, HLA-DR4 occurs in 69% to 70% of seropositive individuals with RA as compared to 25% to 30% of nondiseased persons. HLA-DR1 is found in the majority of HLA-DR4-negative patients and is most strongly associated with this disease in other ethnic groups (e.g., Ashkenzai, South Asians). The presence of HLA-DR4 has also been observed in a high proportion of patients with Sjögren syndrome and multiple sclerosis. The HLA-B27 allele is associated with other autoimmune disorders, such as ankylosing spondylitis, psoriatic arthritis, Reiter's syndrome, reactive arthritis, and inflammatory bowel disease.

195–D

Eighty percent of patients with RA are positive for rheumatoid factor, which is composed of autoantibodies to the Fc portion of IgG molecules. Despite the extremely strong association of rheumatoid factor with RA, a number of other diseases may have positive rheumatoid factor titers, including bacterial endocarditis, tuberculosis, syphilis, kala-azar, viral infections, intravenous drug abuse, and cirrhosis.

196–D

Initial therapy in RA includes adequate rest, anti-inflammatory therapy, and joint-mobility exercises. Initial pharmacologic therapy usually involves nonsteroidal anti-inflammatory drugs, steroid therapy if severe, and various "DMARDS"

(disease modifying antirheumatic drugs) including Plaquenil (hydroxychloroquine), gold, penicillamine, sulfasalazine, and minocycline. Methotrexate is the most widely used and effective form of long-term therapy for RA. Immunosuppressive agents such as azathioprine, cyclophosphamide, chlorambucil, and cyclosporine may be used as last-resort medications for severe, unremitting RA, but would not be used initially.

197–D

Data from numerous studies have shown that ACE inhibitors slow the progression of renal failure, independent of their effects on reducing blood pressure, with several types of kidney disease. Multiple studies have shown their efficacy in reducing the risk of progression to diabetic nephropathy in both types I and II DM, especially in the presence of proteinuria. Another study has looked at the efficacy of ACE inhibition in other renal conditions (Maschio G, Albertl D, Janin G, et al. N Engl J Med 1996;334:939–945) and has shown that these medications do seem to slow progression of renal failure in any process where baseline urinary protein excretion is >1 gram in 24 hours. In this study, the beneficial effect of ACE inhibitors seems to be greatest for males, patients with diabetic nephropathy, patients with baseline proteinuria as above, and glomerular disease. A recent meta-analysis (Jafar TH, Schmid CH, Landa M, et al. Ann Intern Med 2001;135:73–87) compiled the studies looking at treatment of non-diabetic renal disease with ACE inhibitors and found that the relative risk for developing ESRD for these patients was 0.69 in the ACE inhibitor group compared to those treated with other hypertensives, even when adjusting for blood pressure control. This review confirmed that the patients with greater urinary protein excretion at baseline (>0.5 g/day in this particular analysis) showed the greatest benefit from ACE inhibitor therapy.

198–C

Calcium channel blockers have also been shown to slow the progression to renal failure in diabetic nephropathy but are second-line therapy after ACE inhibitors (Tarnow L, Rossing P, Jensen C, et al. Diabetes Care 2000;23:1725–1730). The angiotensin II (AT-II) receptor antagonists (such as losartan) delay the progression of renal failure in animal models of diabetic nephropathy, but human trials are still underway (The Irbesartan Type II Diabetic Nephropathy Trial, in Nephrol

Dialysis Transplant 2000;15:487–497). Some authors suggest using combinations of ACE inhibitors and calcium channel antagonists, and even ACE inhibitors and AT-II receptor blockers, to slow the progression of diabetic nephropathy.

199–B

Erythropoietin (EPO) is a glycoprotein hormone produced primarily by cells of the peritubular capillary endothelium of the kidney and is responsible for the regulation of red blood cell production. Small amounts of the hormone are also synthesized in liver hepatocytes of healthy adults. EPO production is stimulated by reduced oxygen content in the renal arterial circulation. In the presence of renal failure, EPO production decreases, which is largely responsible for the anemia seen in ESRD. Anemia may occur with reductions of renal function of 30% to 50% of normal values, and tends to be progressive. When measured in ESRD, EPO levels are typically within the "normal" range of 15–30 mU/mL, which reflects an inappropriately low response to anemia.

The gene encoding human EPO was cloned in 1985, ultimately leading to the ability to produce recombinant EPO (called rHuEPO). This agent is licensed for use in the treatment of the anemia of renal failure and is usually given subcutaneously three times a week at doses of 50–75 U/kg with a target hematocrit of 33% to 36%. Supplemental iron is often required in patients taking rHuEPO.

200–A

Calcitriol is the active vitamin D metabolite (1,25-dihydroxyvitamin D), whose synthesis is completed by an enzyme produced in the kidney. Calcitriol increases intestinal absorption of calcium and helps suppress PTH production by the parathyroid gland. The reduction of calcitriol production that occurs in advanced renal disease leads to decreased intestinal calcium absorption and the hypocalcemia of kidney disease. This hypocalcemia acts to stimulate PTH production, in an attempt to mobilize calcium from bone. In addition, nephron loss leads to decreased phosphate excretion, resulting in hyperphosphatemia. Phosphate binds directly to calcium, leads to a reduction of calcitriol production by the kidney, and also leads to stimulation of PTH production. This secondary hyperparathyroidism of advanced renal failure leads to increased bone turnover and bone loss, a condition called renal osteodystrophy. Proper supplementation of calcium and vitamin D, along with administration of phosphate binders, help preclude this complication of renal failure.

INDEX

Page numbers followed by *f* refer to figures; page numbers followed by *t* refer to tables.

A-a gradient, 3, 106
Abbreviations, x–xii
Abdomen
  acute, 119
  pain in, 34–55
    foot drop with, 54
    vomiting with, 44–45, 119
  swollen, 52–53, 121–122
ACE. *See* Angiotensin-converting
    enzyme inhibitors
Acetaminophen overdose, 50–51,
    51*f*, 121
N-acetylcysteine, 121
Acquired immunodeficiency syndrome.
    See AIDS
Acute lymphocytic leukemia (ALL), 82
Acute myelogenous leukemia (AML), 82
Adrenal insufficiency, 62–63, 124–125
Adrenocorticotropic hormone (ACTH),
    63, 124–125
Aeromonas hydrophila, 40
AIDS. *See also* HIV disease
  candidiasis in, 46–47, 47*f*, 119–120
  colitis in, 42
  infections of, 120*t*
  pneumonia and, 111
  substance abuse and, 19
  tuberculosis and, 72, 73*t*, 127
Alcohol abuse. *See also* Substance
    abuse
  arrhythmia with, 22
  gout and, 92
  pancreatitis from, 120
α_1-antitrypsin deficiency, 106
Alveolar-arterial (A-a) gradient, 3, 106
Amiodarone, 16–17, 16*f*, 17*f*, 108–109,
    109*t*
Amoxicillin
  rash with, 133
  for sinusitis, 128
Amphotericin B, 120
Ampicillin
  for cholecystitis, 117
  for diarrhea, 41
  for meningitis, 128
Amyloidosis
  arthritis and, 99*t*
  cardiomyopathy from, 108
  nephropathy from, 135
  thrombocytopenia and, 87*t*
Anemia, 84–85, 131
  classification of, 84
  iron deficiency, 84, 131
  leukemia and, 130
  nephropathy and, 137
  SLE and, 134*t*
Aneurysm
  aortic, 27, 48
  mycotic, 19

Angina
  aortic stenosis with, 28, 29*t*
  postinfarction, 115
  unstable, 24–25, 25*f*, 112
Angiotensin-converting enzyme (ACE)
    inhibitors
  for aortic stenosis, 113–114
  for CHF, 108
  diabetes and, 65, 125
  for myocardial infarction, 114–115
  for nephrotic syndrome, 135
  for renal failure, 136–137
Angiotensin II receptor antagonists,
    136–137
Anion gap, 56, 123
Ankylosing spondylitis, 136
Anticardiolipin antibody, 106
Anticoagulants, 105–106
  for angina, 112
  for atrial fibrillation, 111–112
  for CHF, 108
  nephropathy and, 135
  thrombocytopenia and, 106, 129*t*
Antiphospholipid antibody syndrome, 105*t*
Antithrombin deficiency, 105*t*, 106
Aorta
  aneurysm of, 27, 48
  coarctation of, 113
  dissection of, 26–27, 26*f*, 38, 48, 113,
    115
Aortic valve
  replacement of, 113–114
  stenosis of, 28–29, 29*t*, 114
    chest pain and, 32
    treatment for, 113–114
Aortography, 113
Appendicitis, 38
Arrhythmia
  myocardial infarction and, 115
  shortness of breath with, 22–23, 22*f*
Arthritis, 92, 94
  causes of, 99*t*
  psoriatic, 99*t*, 136
  rheumatoid, 13, 98–99, 135–136
    classification of, 135*t*
    interstitial lung disease and, 109*t*
    treatment of, 136
Asbestosis, 109*t*
Ascites, 52–53, 121–122
Aspirin
  for angina, 25
  asthma and, 4
  for atrial fibrillation, 111
  for gout, 133
  for myocardial infarction, 31, 115
  nephrotic syndrome and, 135
Asthma, 4–5, 105–106
  flow-volume loop for, 5*f*
AT-II receptor antagonists, 136–137
Atovaquone, 120*t*
Atrial fibrillation, 22–23, 22*f*, 111–112
Azathioprine, 120, 136
Azithromycin, 120*t*, 129

Bacillus cereus, 40
Bagassosis, 109*t*
Barrett's esophagus, 116
Berylliosis, 109*t*
Beta-blockers
  for aortic stenosis, 114
  for atrial fibrillation, 111
  for CHF, 108
  for COPD, 106
  for myocardial infarction, 114–115
Bird breeder's lung, 109*t*
Bismuth subsalicylate, 118
Bleeding gums, 80–81
Bleomycin, 87*t*
Borrelia burgdorferi, 92
Bowel. *See also* Inflammatory bowel
    disease
  infarcted, 119
  ischemic, 44–45, 48, 119
Breast cancer, 60–61, 60*f*, 61*t*, 124
  screening for, 68–69, 126
Bronchiolitis obliterans, 109*t*
Brucellosis, 88
Buffalo hump, 62
Buprenorphine, 110
Butterfly rash, 94*f*, 134

Calcitriol, 137
Calcium channel blockers
  aortic stenosis and, 113–114
  for CHF, 108
  renal failure and, 136–137
Campylobacter jejuni, 40, 42, 118
Candidiasis, esophageal, 46–47, 47*f*,
    119–120, 120*f*
Cardiomyopathy
  atrial fibrillation and, 111
  categories of, 108
  CHF with, 14–15, 108
  hypertrophic, 32
Cefotaxime
  for meningitis, 128
  for pneumonia, 111
Ceftriaxone
  for meningitis, 128
  for pharyngitis, 129
  for pneumonia, 111
Cephalosporins
  for cholecystitis, 117
  for pharyngitis, 129
  for sinusitis, 128
Cerebrospinal fluid (CSF), 128
Ceruloplasmin, 121
Cervical cancer screening, 68
Charcot's triad, 117
Chest pain, 24–33
  non-cardiac, 32–33, 115
  pleuritic, 21
  shortness of breath with, 24–25
CHF. *See* Congestive heart failure
Chlamydia pneumoniae, 111
Chlamydia trachomatis, 129
Chlorambucil, 136

INDEX

Cholangitis, 38–39, 117–118
Cholecystitis, 38, 48
Cholesterol
  calculation of, 70–71, 127
  treatment for, 126
Chronic fatigue syndrome, 98
Chronic obstructive pulmonary disease
  (COPD), 8–9, 106–107
  stages of, 8t
Churg-Strauss syndrome, 109t, 122
Chylothorax, 13
Ciprofloxacin
  for diarrhea, 41, 118
  for meningitis, 128
  pneumococci and, 111
Cirrhosis
  ascites with, 52–53, 121–122
  pleural effusions and, 13
  rheumatoid factor and, 136
Cisplatin, 87t
Clostridium dificile
  colitis from, 19
  diarrhea from, 42–43
Clotting factors, 121
CMV. See Cytomegalovirus
Coal workers' pneumoconiosis, 109t
Colchicine, 133–134
Colitis, 42–43
  pseudomembranous, 119
  ulcerative, 42, 106, 118–119
Colon cancer screening, 69, 126
Colonoscopy, 68, 126
Community-acquired pneumonia (CAP),
  20–21, 20f, 110–111. See also
  Pneumonia
Congestive heart failure (CHF)
  aortic stenosis and, 28, 29t
  atrial fibrillation and, 111
  cardiomyopathy with, 14–15, 108
  hyperthyroidism and, 126
  pleural effusions and, 13, 107
  pulmonary edema with, 10
  right-sided, 6
  thrombotic syndromes with, 105t
  underlying diseases of, 14–15
COPD. See Chronic obstructive
  pulmonary disease
Coronary heart disease (CHD)
  angina and, 24
  cholesterol and, 70–71, 70t, 127
  diabetes and, 125
  myocardial infarction and, 30
  risks for, 32, 71, 127
Cor pulmonale, 105
  asthma and, 5
Corticosteroids. See Steroids
Cortisol, 63, 124
Coxsackie A virus, 78
Crohn's disease, 42–43, 118–119
  treatment of, 119
Cryoglobulinemia, 91t
Cryptosporidiosis, 40
Cushing's syndrome, 62–63, 124–125
Cyclophosphamide
  for arthritis, 136
  for polyarteritis nodosa, 122
Cyclosporine
  for arthritis, 136
  for ulcerative colitis, 119
Cytomegalovirus (CMV)
  colitis from, 42
  esophagitis and, 46
  HIV infection and, 88

Dapsone, 120t
Dexamethasone, 125
Diabetes mellitus, 64–65, 65t, 125
  nephropathy from, 135
  renal failure with, 100–101, 101t
  risks for, 125
  tuberculosis and, 73t
Diabetic ketoacidosis (DKA), 56–57,
  122–123
Diarrhea
  fever with, 42–43
  traveler's, 40–41, 118, 118f
Diazoxide, 107
DIC. See Disseminated intravascular
  coagulation
Digitalis, 114
Digoxin
  for atrial fibrillation, 111
  for CHF, 108
Diltiazem
  for atrial fibrillation, 111
  for CHF, 108
Discoid lupus erythematosus, 134
Disseminated intravascular coagulation
  (DIC), 105t, 129t
  leukemia and, 130
  thrombocytopenia and, 87t
Diuretics. See also Thiazides
  for aortic stenosis, 114
  ascites and, 122
  for CHF, 108
DMARDS, 136
Doxorubicin, 108
Doxycycline, 129
Drug abuse. See Substance abuse
Duke criteria for endocarditis, 110
Dysfibrinogenemia, 106

Eaton-Lambert syndrome, 113
Eclampsia, 87t
Edema
  peripheral, 96, 134–135
  pulmonary, 135
Ehlers-Danlos syndrome, 113
Electrocardiography (ECG)
  angina on, 25f
  atrial fibrillation on, 22f
  hypercalcemia and, 124
  hyperthyroidism on, 66f, 67
  myocardial infarction on, 30f, 114
  pulmonary embolism and, 105
Embolism, pulmonary, 2–3, 2f, 6, 105
  chest pain with, 115
  endocarditis and, 110
  pleural effusions and, 13
  risks for, 105t
Emphysema, 106
Empty sella syndrome, 123t
Empyema, 12–13, 12f, 107–108
Enalaprilat, 107
Encephalopathy, hepatic, 122
Endocarditis, 74
  aortic stenosis and, 114
  glomerulonephritis and, 91t
  nephrotic syndrome and, 135
  rash with, 94
  rheumatoid factor and, 136
  substance abuse and, 19, 110
Entamoeba histolytica, 40, 42
Enterococcus faecalis, 122
Environmental hazards, 109t
Epigastric pain, 48–49
Epstein-Barr virus (EBV), 88, 133

Erythropoietin, 137
Escherichia coli
  diarrhea from, 40, 42
  hemolytic-uremic syndrome
    and, 131
  peritonitis from, 122
Esmolol, 107, 111
Esophagus
  Barrett's, 116
  candidiasis of, 46–47, 47f, 119–120,
    120t
  spasm of, 115
Estrogens
  hypercalcemia from, 61t
  pancreatitis from, 120
Exercise treadmill testing, 114–115

Factor V Leiden, 105t, 106
Familial hypocalciuric hypercalcemia,
  61t
Farmer's lung, 109t
Fever
  diarrhea with, 42–43
  headache with, 74–75
  rash with, 88–89
  right upper quadrant pain with,
    38–39
  shortness of breath with, 12–13, 12f,
    107–108
    cough and, 20–21, 20f, 110–111
  swollen abdomen with, 52–53
Fibrinolytic disorders, 105t
Fibromyalgia, 135–136
Flow-volume loops, 5f
Fluconazole, 119
Fluoroquinolones
  for cholecystitis, 117
  for diarrhea, 41, 118
  for meningitis, 128
  for peritonitis, 122
  for pneumonia, 111
  for sinusitis, 128
Focal segmental glomerulosclerosis
  (FSGS), 135
Folate, 84
Foot drop, 54
Friedewald equation, 71
Furosemide, 120

Gall bladder disease, 38–39, 117–118,
  120
Gastroenteritis, 44
Gastroesophageal reflux disease (GERD),
  34–35, 35f, 115–116
  chest pain with, 32
  risks for, 115–116
  stages of, 116t
  treatment of, 116
Gastrointestinal bleed, 36–37, 116–117
Gaucher disease, 109t
Gemfibrozil, 126
Gentamicin, 128
GERD. See Gastroesophageal reflux
  disease
Giant cell arteritis, 54
Giardia lamblia, 40, 118f
Glomerulonephritis
  poststreptococcal, 90–91, 90f, 133
  renal failure from, 101t
  tests for, 91t
Glomerulonephropathy, 135
Glucocorticoids, 62–63. See also
  Steroids

Glucose measurements, 65t
Goiter, 126
Gonorrhea, 88. See also Sexually
   transmitted diseases
   arthritis from, 92, 99t, 133
   pharyngitis from, 129
   proctitis from, 42
   rash with, 94
Goodpasture syndrome, 91t, 109t
Gout, 92–93, 99t, 133–134
Graves disease, 66–67
Guaifenesin, 128
Gums, bleeding, 80–81

Haemophilus influenzae, 111
Hampton's hump, 3
Hashimoto's thyroiditis, 58–59, 123t
HBV. See Hepatitis B virus
Heartburn, 34
Helicobacter pylori, 116
HELLP syndrome, 87t
Hemangioma, 87t
Hematemesis, 36–37, 116–117
Hematochezia, 36
Hematologic disorders, 80–89. See also
   specific types, e.g., Anemia
Hemochromatosis, 108
Hemoglobin A1C, 65t
Hemolytic-uremic syndrome (HUS), 129t
   thrombocytopenia and, 87, 131
Henoch-Schönlein purpura, 91t
Heparin, 105. See also Anticoagulants
   for angina, 112
   thrombocytopenia and, 106, 129t
Heparin cofactor II deficiency, 105t
Hepatitis A virus (HAV), 88
Hepatitis B virus (HBV), 38, 88
   arthritis and, 99t
   isoniazid and, 127–128
   nephrotic syndrome and, 135
   polyarteritis nodosa and, 122
   substance abuse and, 19
Hepatitis C virus (HCV)
   ascites and, 52–53
   liver failure and, 121
   nephrotic syndrome and, 135
   substance abuse and, 19
Hepatitis D virus, 121
Hepatolenticular degeneration, 121
Hermansky-Pudlak syndrome, 109t
Heroin. See also Substance abuse
   anemia and, 84
   empyema and, 12
   Graves disease and, 66
   nephrotic syndrome and, 135
Herpes simplex virus (HSV)
   esophagitis and, 46
   HIV infection and, 88
   pharyngitis and, 178
Hirudin, 105
Histiocytosis X, 109t
HIV disease, 88–89, 131–133
   arthritis and, 92
   candidiasis in, 46–47, 47f, 119–120
   CD4 counts in, 132f
   colitis in, 42
   infections of, 120t
   nephropathy from, 101t
   nephrotic syndrome and, 135
   pneumonia and, 111
   substance abuse and, 19
   symptoms of, 132t
   thrombocytopenia and, 131

treatment of, 133
   tuberculosis and, 72, 73t, 127
Hodgkin disease, 135
Holiday heart, 22
Hormonal imbalances, 56–67
HSV. See Herpes simplex virus
Human herpes virus-6, 88
Human immunodeficiency virus.
   See HIV disease
HUS. See Hemolytic-uremic syndrome
Hydralazine, 107
Hydrocortisone, 125
Hydroxychloroquine, 136
Hypercalcemia, 60–61, 60f, 124
   causes of, 61t
   cortisol and, 62
Hypercholesterolemia, 70–71, 127
   treatment of, 71, 127
Hypercoagulability, 3, 6, 105t
   hypertension and, 106
Hyperhomocystinemia, 105t
Hyperparathyroidism, 61t
Hyperphosphatemia, 137
Hypertension
   arrhythmia with, 22
   cholesterol and, 70–71
   diabetes and, 125
   pulmonary, 6–7, 106
   renal failure from, 101t
   shortness of breath with, 10–11, 107
   thrombocytopenia and, 87t
   treatment of, 126
Hypertensive emergency, 10–11, 107
Hypertensive urgency, 107
Hyperthyroidism, 66–67, 66f, 125–126.
   See also Thyroid disorders
   apathetic, 126
Hypoalbuminemia, 134
Hypokalemia, 105
Hypothyroidism, 58–59, 123–124. See
   also Thyroid disorders
   anemia and, 84
   types of, 123t

Idiopathic thrombocytopenic purpura
   (ITP), 80–81, 129–130, 129t
Immunizations, adult, 68
Inflammatory bowel disease (IBD),
   42–44, 118–119, 136
Interstitial lung disease (ILD), 16f, 17f
   categories of, 109t
Ipratopium bromide, 106
Ischemic bowel, 44–45, 48, 119
Isoniazid
   regimen for, 127t
   side effects of, 127–128
Itraconazole, 119

Kala-azar, 136
Kasabach-Merritt syndrome, 87t
Ketoconazole, 120
Klebsiella pneumoniae, 111
Knee, gouty, 92
Kussmaul respirations, 56

Labetalol, 107
Lansoprazole, 116
Lanugo, 62
Legionellosis, 111
Leptospirosis, 88
Leucovorin, 120t
Leukemia, 54, 82–83, 124, 130–131
   tuberculosis and, 73t

Levofloxacin, 111
Listeria monocytogenes, 128
Lithium, 61t
Liver
   abscess of, 38
   metastasis to, 60f
Loeffler's endocarditis, 108
Losartan, 136
Low-density lipoprotein (LDL), 70–71,
   70t, 127
Lumbar puncture, 74
Lungs
   edema of, 10
   interstitial disease of, 16–17, 16f,
     17f, 109t
   metastasis to, 60f
   scan of, 105
   white, 16–17
Lupus anticoagulant, 106
Lyme disease, 92, 94
Lymphoma, 54, 124
   tuberculosis and, 73t

Malaria, 88
Mallory-Weiss tear
   chest pain with, 32
   hematemesis and, 117
Marfan syndrome, 113
Melena, 36
Membranoproliferative
   glomerulonephropathy (MPGN),
   135
Meningitis, 74–75, 128
Meningococcemia, 88
Metabolic acidosis, 56
Metformin, 65, 125
Methadone, 110
Methicillin resistance, 110
Methimazole, 125–126
Metoprolol, 111
Metronidazole
   for cholecystitis, 117
   for diarrhea, 118
Microangiopathic hemolytic anemia
   (MAHA), 86, 87t
Milk-alkali syndrome, 61t
Minimal change disease (MCD), 135
Minocycline, 136
Mitomycin C, 87t
Mononucleosis, 78
Moraxella catarrhalis, 111
Mortality, causes of, 107
Moxifloxacin, 111
MPGN, 135
MUDPILES, 56, 119
Multiple myeloma, 101
Multiple sclerosis, 136
Mycobacterium avium complex
   (MAC), 120t
Mycobacterium avium-intracellulare
   (MAI), 46, 120
Mycobacterium tuberculosis. See
   Tuberculosis
Mycoplasma pneumoniae, 111
Myeloproliferative disorders, 105t
Myocardial infarction (MI), 30–31, 30f,
   114–115
   Q wave, 30f, 31, 112, 114
   types of, 114
Myocarditis, 112

Nafcillin, 110
Necrotizing fasciitis, 19

INDEX

Neisseria gonorrhoeae. *See also* Sexually
    transmitted diseases
    arthritis from, 92, 99t, 133
    pharyngitis from, 129
    proctitis from, 42
    rash with, 94
Neisseria meningitides, 128
Nephritis, 91t
Nephropathy. *See also* Renal failure
    diabetic, 64, 100–101, 136–137
    membranous, 135
Nephrotic syndrome, 96–97, 134–135
    definition of, 134
    pleural effusions and, 13
    thrombotic syndromes with, 105t
Neurofibromatosis, 109t
Neuroleptic malignant syndrome, 74
Neuropathy
    diabetic, 64–65, 125
    isoniazid and, 127–128
Neutropenia, 130–131
Niemann-Pick disease, 109t
Nifedipine, 107
Nitroglycerin, 32, 107, 115
Nitroprusside, 107
Nomogram, Rumack-Matthew, 50–51,
    51f
Non-Hodgkin lymphoma, 124
Norwalk virus, 40
Nosebleed, 82

Odynophagia, 46, 119
Omeprazole, 116
Opportunistic infections, 120t
Oral contraceptive risks, 3, 105t
Otitis media, 128
Ovarian cancer, 124
Overdose, acetaminophen, 50–51, 51f,
    121
Oxacillin, 110
Oxymetazoline, 128

Paget disease, 61t
Palpitations, 14f, 22–23, 22f, 111–112
Pamidronate, 61
Pancreatitis, 38
    acute, 48–49, 49f, 120–121
    pleural effusions and, 13
Papanicolaou smears, 68
Parathyroid carcinoma, 61t
Paroxysmal nocturnal hemoglobinuria,
    105t
PCP. *See Pneumocystis carinii*
    pneumonia
Penicillamine, 135–136
Penicillin, 133
Pentamidine
    pancreatitis from, 120
    for PCP, 120t
Peptic ulcer, 38
Percutaneous transluminal coronary
    angioplasty (PTCA), 112, 114
Peritonitis, 52–53, 119, 122
Pharyngitis, 78–79, 88, 129
    glomerulonephritis after, 90–91, 133
Phenylephrine, 128
Phenylpropanolamine, 128
Photosensitivity, 134t
Pituitary tumor, 123t
Plesimonas shigelloides, 40
Pleural effusions, 12–13, 107
Pneumoconiosis, 109t

Pneumocystis carinii pneumonia
    (PCP), 111
    prevention of, 120t
Pneumonia
    arrhythmia with, 22
    community-acquired, 20–21, 20f,
        110–111
    empyema from, 107
    eosinophilic, 109t
    interstitial, 17, 109t
    tuberculosis and, 111
Pneumothorax
    after thoracentesis, 12
    treatment of, 108
    from ventilation, 106
Polyarteritis nodosa, 54–55, 122
    thrombocytopenia and, 87t
Polycystic kidney disease, 101t
Polycystic ovary disease, 125
Poststreptococcal glomerulonephritis
    (PSGN), 90–91, 90f, 133
Pravastatin, 71
Prednisone, 9
Preeclampsia, 87t
Probenecid, 133
Propranolol, 125
Propylthiouracil, 67, 125–126
Prostacyclin, 106
Prostate serum antigen (PSA) test, 68
Protein C deficiency, 105t, 106
Protein S deficiency, 106
Proteinuria, 134
Proton pump inhibitors, 116
Pseudoephedrine, 128
Pseudogout, 92, 99t, 134
Pseudothrombocytopenia, 129t
PSGN (poststreptococcal
    glomerulonephritis), 90–91
PTCA (percutaneous transluminal
    coronary angioplasty), 112, 114
Pulmonary edema, 10
Pulmonary embolism, 2–3, 2f, 6, 105
    arrhythmia with, 22
    chest pain with, 115
    endocarditis and, 110
    pleural effusions and, 13
    risks for, 105t
Pulmonary fibrosis, 16–17, 16f, 17f,
    108–109
Pulmonary hypertension, 6–7, 106
Pulsus parvus et tardus, 114
P-wave pulmonale, 105
Pyrazinamide (PZA), 127f
Pyridoxine, 128
Pyrimethamine, 120t

Q wave myocardial infarction, 30f, 31,
    112, 114

Ranson's score, 120–121
Reiter's syndrome, 99t, 136
Renal failure. *See also* Nephropathy
    ACE inhibitors and, 136–137
    acute, 90–91, 90f, 91t, 133
    chronic, 100–101, 136–137
        causes of, 101t
    hypercalcemia from, 61t
    leukemia and, 130
    nephrotic syndrome and, 135
    tuberculosis and, 73t
Respiratory acidosis, 4–5
Respiratory alkalosis, 105

Reticulocytosis, 84
Retinopathy, diabetic, 64–65
Rhabdomyolysis, 61t
Rheumatoid arthritis, 13, 98–99,
    135–136. *See also* Arthritis
    causes of, 99t
    classification of, 135t
    interstitial lung disease and, 109t
    treatment of, 136
Rifabutin, 120t
Rifampin
    for meningitis, 128
    for TB, 127t
Roseola, 88
Rotavirus, 40
Rubella, 99t
Rumack-Matthew nomogram, 50–51, 51f

Salmonellosis, 40, 42
Sarcoidosis
    arthritis and, 99t
    cardiomyopathy from, 108
    hypothyroidism with, 123t
    interstitial lung disease with, 109t
    pleural effusions with, 13
Schistocytes, 86f
Scleroderma
    interstitial lung disease and, 109t
    thrombocytopenia and, 87t
Screening tests, 68–69, 126
Serum-ascites albumin gradient (SAAG),
    121–122
Sexually transmitted diseases (STDs), 88
    aortic dissection from, 113
    gout and, 92, 133
    proctitis from, 42
    rash with, 94
Shigellosis, 40, 42
Shortness of breath (SOB), 2–23
    acute, 2–3, 2f, 105
    chest pain with, 24–25
    chronic, 6–9, 8t, 106–107
    fever with, 12–13, 12f, 107–108
        cough and, 20–21, 20f, 110–111
    hypertension with, 10–11, 107
    palpitations with, 14f, 22–23, 22f,
        111–112
    renal failure with, 100–101
    sunken cheeks with, 56–57
Sigmoidoscopy, 68, 126
Silicosis, 73t, 109t
Simvastatin, 65
Sinusitis, 76–77
    treatment of, 128–129
Sjögren syndrome, 99t, 136
Skip lesions, 18
SOB. *See* Shortness of breath
Solu-Medrol, 106
Spironolactone, 108
Spontaneous bacterial peritonitis (SBP),
    52–53, 122
Stanford classification, 27
Staphylococcal infections
    arthritis from, 99t
    diarrhea from, 40
    pneumonia from, 111
    substance abuse and, 19, 109–110
STDs. *See* Sexually transmitted diseases
Steroids
    adrenal insufficiency and, 62
    for asthma, 105–106
    for COPD, 8–9

for gout, 133–134
for hyperthyroidism, 125
for inflammatory bowel disease, 119
for polyarteritis nodosa, 122
Streptococcal infections
antibodies to, 133
arthritis from, 99t
meningitis from, 75
peritonitis from, 122
pharyngeal, 78–79, 129
pneumonia from, 111
substance abuse and, 19
ST segment elevations, 112
Subarachnoid hemorrhage, 74
Substance abuse. See also specific types,
e.g., Alcohol abuse
anemia and, 84
empyema from, 12
Graves disease and, 66
infections from, 18–19, 18f, 109–110
nephrotic syndrome and, 135
rheumatoid factor and, 136
Sulfasalazine, 136
Sulfonamides, 120
Swelling, 90–101
Syncope, 28–29, 29t
Syphilis. See also Sexually transmitted
diseases
aortic dissection from, 113
rash with, 94
rheumatoid factor and, 136
secondary, 88
Systemic lupus erythematosus (SLE),
94–95, 134
arthritis and, 99t
butterfly rash of, 94f, 134
classification of, 134t
glomerulonephritis with, 91t
interstitial lung disease and, 109t
pleural effusions with, 13
thrombocytopenia and, 87t, 130

Takayasu's arteritis, 54, 122
Tetanus
immunizations for, 68
substance abuse and, 19
Tetracycline
pancreatitis from, 120
for pneumonia, 111

Thalassemia, 84
Theophylline, 61t
Thiazides. See also Diuretics
gout and, 133–134
hypercalcemia from, 61t
pancreatitis from, 120
Thoracentesis, 12
Thrombocytopenia
classification of, 129t
disorders of, 87t
heparin-induced, 106
Thrombolytic therapy, 31, 114–115
Thrombomodulin dysfunction, 105t
Thrombophlebitis, 105
septic, 19, 110
Thrombotic syndromes, 3, 6
hypertension and, 106
risks for, 105t
Thrombotic thrombocytopenic purpura
(TTP), 86–87, 86f, 87t, 129t, 131
Thyroid disorders, 58–59, 66–67, 66f,
123–126, 123t
anemia and, 84
arrhythmia with, 22
Thyroid-stimulating hormone (TSH),
58–59
Thyroid storm, 67, 125
Thyrotropin-releasing hormone (TRH),
58
Thyroxine (T$_4$), 58, 125
Tobacco use
COPD and, 106
hypercoagulability and, 105t
oral contraceptives and, 3
Toxoplasmosis, 88, 120t
Tracheomalacia, 106
Transjugular intrahepatic portosystemic
shunt (TIPS), 122
Triiodothyronine (T$_3$), 58, 125
Trimethoprim-sulfamethoxazole
for diarrhea, 41
for opportunistic infections, 120t
for peritonitis, 122
for sinusitis, 128
Trousseau syndrome, 105
Tuberculosis (TB), 120
active vs. latent, 72
arthritis and, 92
hypercalcemia with, 61t

pneumonia and, 111
reaction to, 72–73, 127–128
rheumatoid factor and, 136
risks for, 73t
treatment of, 127t
T wave inversions, 112

Ulcerative colitis, 42, 106, 118
treatment of, 119
Upper respiratory tract infection (URI)
asthma and, 4
sinusitis after, 76
U.S. Preventive Services Task Force
(USPSTF), 68

Valproic acid, 120
Vancomycin
for endocarditis, 110
for meningitis, 128
for pneumonia, 111
Vasculitis, 54–55, 122
Ventilation, complications of, 106
Ventilation-perfusion scan, 3, 105
Verapamil, 108
Vibrio parahaemolyticus, 40
Virchow triad, 3
Vitamin A, 61t
Vitamin B$_6$, 128
Vitamin B$_{12}$
anemia and, 84
metformin and, 125
Vitamin D, 61t, 137
Vitamin K, 121

Warfarin, 105–106. See also
Anticoagulants
for atrial fibrillation, 111–112
nephropathy and, 135
Waters view, 76
Wegener granulomatosis, 54, 109t, 122
sinusitis and, 76
test for, 91t
thrombocytopenia and, 87t
Wellness exam, 68–69, 126
Westermark sign, 3
Wilson's disease, 121
Winter's formula, 56–57

Yersinia enterocolitica, 40, 42